Contents

Acknowledgments

As with many things in life, behind the scene workers never have their true worth and value recognised but without their valuable contribution things would simply not get done. To them we are immensely grateful and owe a debt.

To Mr. Alun Jones, for production and management of the photographic illustrations in this book. He is a man who accepts other people's failings and quietly compensates for them by his own efforts.

All projects require a link between the different contributors and facets. It has been Ms Janet Morris, Mrs Erica Wilkinson and Mrs Judy Harris upon whom we have relied to maintain effective and efficient communications, their skill in negotiation and politics has taught us much.

To Marie Carter for her patience in proof reading this edition.

To all our teachers, both past and present, who although not formally recognised at the beginning of chapters, know by their own efforts that much of what is written is based upon their teaching and wisdom.

And finally to Professor James Richardson, whose drive, enthusiasm and humour is infectious. He is a man who understands that encouragement and support are much more vital and productive than a big stick!

No amount of reading is as good as practical teaching. Oswestry runs a series of courses focussed on Orthopaedic education. A clinical examination course is run by the authors of this book and others, currently 3 times a year here at Oswestry. **BOOK WELL AHEAD !!!**

Professor James Richardson.
July 2006.

Introduction

The final part of the FRCS examination has been described as an exit exam confirming the completion of the candidates' training. The exam was first instigated in 1987. During the 19 years it has been running, the format has evolved and continues to develop. One area that has remained constant is the clinical long and short cases, a format familiar to most candidates from Medical School days.

The pass rate has undergone a process of evolution. In the early days, the pass rates were higher than those experienced now. Whether this describes changes in candidates' ability, training or the demands of the examiners is unclear. As with the driving test, a candidate may feel they can drive a car but needs to display this ability to the examiner and convince them. There are set routines of mirror, signal and manoeuvre, which need to be demonstrated to confirm the candidate's ability. You may feel that you can examine patients, after all you have seen hundreds of patients in clinic over the years, but the examination in a busy outpatients clinic will be different from that in the FRCS (Orth).

This book is designed to help you to form a routine in clinical examination that even under the stress of exam conditions you can perform, allowing your concentration to be focused on the findings rather than what to do next.

There really is no genuine alternative to repeated examination of patients. This is a much more productive and reinforcing experience if performed under the critical eyes of colleagues and seniors. To have a "running mate" in the preparation for the exam is an advantage and to have a consultant cadre interested in teaching, together with the preparation for the exam, is a real ace in your pocket. Seek out help, remember no-one should be an island. There are many areas that are similar in the clinical examination of the different joints.

These are dealt with in this section to avoid repetition throughout the subsequent chapters.

There really should be no need for this section to be discussed but apparently it does. It is important to remember that you are trying to join a club and, as such, appearing like the other members often is the first hurdle.

A sober dress sense, clean, ironed and polished presentation is what is required.

Politeness to both examiner and patients is essential.

Introduce yourself, offer a handshake, but be careful not to hurt the patient with a rheumatoid hand, and ask for permission to examine.

These actions show your concern and respect for patients, and so confirm your competence. However being "Tim nice but dim" or arrogant and brusque will not help your cause. Remember to be careful with your language. It can appear condescending to refer to elderly people as "my dear" but equally so a less formal approach is important with children.

There are two styles of presentation, the "say as you go along and summarise at the end" or " save it up and surprise them at the end". There are advantages and disadvantages with both. The former can sometimes be a distraction, as John Wayne is reported to have said "You want me to walk and talk at the same time! " The latter can lead to an awkward silence that is uncomfortable for all present. The right choice is dependent upon your character and what you feel most comfortable with, practice is the only way to tell which one suits you. We recommend the former though!

General Principles of Examination

Many things by being familiar often pass without comment. The presence of a walking stick, calliper or SOS bracelet may affect decisions regarding management and so deserve comment. Exposure is important to allow an adequate examination but always respect the patient's modesty. It is not unreasonable to comment how you would normally expose a very timid patient and await the examiners lead. Watching the patient undress can give many clues to upper limb function just as watching the patient walking into the examination room can reveal a diagnostic gait. Individual joint examination dictates how you and the patient interact. It is difficult to predict how large the room in your exam will be, so be prepared to adapt as necessary.

The use of tools and gadgets in the clinical has apparently caused humour to examiners in the past. Some candidates have arrived requiring a Sherpa to carry tendon hammers, neurological needles, tuning forks etc. You cannot make up for a lack of confidence or ability by having equipment. Any items that are genuinely needed will be provided. The only exceptions to this rule are a goniometer, a tape measure and a pen. It may seem pernickety but to actually measure the range of movement with a goniometer shows that you recognise that care and accuracy are important in the assessment of a patient.

Inspection

A logical pattern must be followed - it is all too easy to miss a subtle sign, particularly on inspection. Pattern recognition is important - a rheumatoid hand can be easily summarised in a few lines.

The examiner may direct you to closer examination of a specific point. If not, continue on with the routine which you normally follow.

Disease patterns will be discussed in each chapter and more guided examination described.

Deformity can be considered related to the overall limb position (i.e. the valgus knee) or to the surrounding soft tissue and bony contours (i.e. an old clavicle fracture). Describe the former and look closely for the latter.

The skin can give you many clues, Afro-Caribbean origin may mean sickle cell disease is a factor in aetiology or anaesthetic assessment.

Previous keloid or hypertrophic scars should draw attention to the need for careful preoperative counselling and planning.

Bruising may indicate a recent injury (unlikely in the examination), warfarin, heparin or steroid intake.

Redness can be indicative of infection but again is unlikely in the exam, but trophic changes due to a chronic condition are common.

Old scars not only indicate previous surgery, injury or sinuses but also affect any future proposed procedure. Obviously we cannot predict with any certainty what operation has been performed through a specific scar but it does narrow the field of choices.

Consideration of plastic surgery procedures is important, in particular, in lower limb reconstruction cases. The position and type of plastic reconstruction again tells a story. This can also dictate the position of any future surgical incisions.

Wasting may be obvious. Quantifying the wasting such as that in the quadriceps is sometimes useful. Specific wasting patterns and resting position can be diagnostic. Do not be afraid to give a spot diagnosis but be prepared to clarify it with further examination. Always have a different diagnosis in the back of your mind.

General Examination

Palpation

Always ask where it hurts. Most of the clues when you palpate are visible in your patient's expression. Keep one eye on their face, if you are beginning to cause discomfort stop, ask the patient and examiner if it is appropriate to continue.

Specific sites of tenderness combined with particular stress tests can be useful in pin pointing the exact area of pathology. This is also the opportunity to ascertain if the skin temperature is the same on both sides, a difference should be commented upon.

As with inspection be methodical.

In particular practice your patter for the description of lumps and bumps (i.e. **S**ite, **S**hape, **S**ize, **S**urface, **S**urrounding tissue, con**S**istency and lymph node**S**).

Circulation should be assessed and recorded as it can effect dramatically how you might manage the patient. The sensory function can be assessed with the MRC score:-

1   Completely absent sensation
2   Presence of deep cutaneous pain
3   Some cutaneous pain and soft touch sensation
4   Two point discrimination
5   Normal

Movement

It is traditional to examine the active movement and complete the passive movement. This is sometimes combined with specific tests and is best appreciated in each individual system. Watch out for pain. Examining the asymptomatic first will provide you with a baseline. The rhythm of movement is sometimes more important than the arc. The effect of moving one joint on another becomes important in hand examination. The ranges of movement quoted are based upon those given in "The Clinical measurement of Joint Motion" by Greene W B and Heckmann J D, ISBN 0-89203-090-9. It should of course be borne in mind that the normal range of motion in a joint reduces quite naturally with age.

Power

The power of muscle contraction needs to be assessed in an accurate manner. This is best described by the MRC scale:-

0   No discernible muscle contraction.
1   A flicker of muscle activity but insufficient to move the joint.
2   Muscle contraction is present but weak and can only move the joint if gravity is eliminated and the limb weight is counterbalanced.
3   Muscle contraction is present and sufficient to move the joint against the force of gravity.
4   Near normal muscle power and ability.
5   Normal.

It is important to qualify if any apparent reduction in muscle strength is caused by pain inhibition. The ultimate test of power in the lower limb should be completed by assessing the gait. A more subtle abnormality may become evident.

Special Tests

The examination is completed by the relevant special tests. This is an opportunity to summarise the findings in your own mind and look for more specific signs.

It is often helpful to think along the lines of a specific condition, these are described in the clinical cases discussed at the end of each chapter.

The clinical relevance of each test can be described as each test is performed or summarised at the end.

Summary

Be polite and courteous.

Do not hurt the patient.

Be systematic.

Be clear and concise in your summary.

Be ready for the onslaught.

Do not give up! (You may have passed a section when you think you have not!)

The Hand and Wrist

Ms Katrina Lewis FRCS, FRCS(Orth),
Consultant Orthopaedic and Hand Surgeon.

Exposure

Expose the whole of the upper limbs including the neck, shoulders and the elbows. Seat the patient so that they are comfortable; consider using a small table to rest the hands on. Ensure that the lighting is good, attention to detail means you will not miss something that it is important.

Inspection

Begin with the hands in the resting position, actively comparing both sides. This needs to be done on both the palmar and dorsal surfaces. Contrast the size and relative dimensions of the digits and hand itself. Hypertrophy of a single digit may be due to Paget's disease, neurofibromatosis (look for café au lait spots) or a local A-V fistula. Other spot diagnoses are Marfan's syndrome presenting with long slender proximal phalanges or the short ring metacarpal of Turner's syndrome.

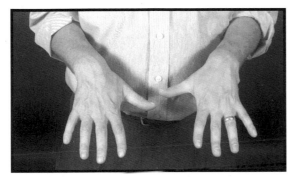 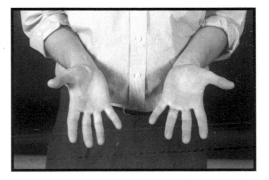

Fig.1 Look carefully at both surfaces of the hand and wrist, observe deformity, scars and muscle wasting.

DEFORMITY & CONTOUR

Describe the resting position and any obvious deformities. This often gives you the diagnosis. A nerve lesion will produce a specific resting position - it maybe worthwhile, if you are sure, to describe the pattern of deformity and give your provisional diagnosis. The examiner may just ask you to confirm your suspicions but always have a different diagnosis in mind just in case you were wrong!

Obviously, if the patient has multiple problems, in particular a rheumatoid hand, the abnormalities will need to be defined individually in context with the whole problem.

A simple statement such as *'This patient has a symmetrical polyarthropathy affecting mainly the proximal joints with.....'* is a good starting point with complex deformities.

Each specific problem may require further examination after the initial findings are presented.

> **Specific finger deformities**
> | | |
> |---|---|
> | Mallet finger | Dupuytrens disease |
> | Swan neck deformity | Syndactaly |
> | Boutonniere deformity | Malunited fracture |
> | Z thumb | |

Do not get bogged down in describing one abnormality in the hand, work through the problems systematically and be guided by the examiner as to which they specifically want to concentrate on. This will be become more important when the special tests are considered.

The Hand and Wrist

Describe any obvious swellings. Hand tumours are a common short case. The examiner then may direct you towards a more specific examination described in the examination of a lump. Fusiform swellings around joints are often rheumatological but you do need to consider unusual causes such as T.B, gout, syphilis or sarcoidosis.

> **Hand Tumours**
> Ganglion
> Mucous cyst
> Giant cell tumour
> Villonodular synovitis
> Bone tumours
> Skin tumours

SKIN & SCARS

Study the nails. At medical school we were all familiar with the causes of clubbing and although not always directly involved with orthopaedic surgery. This observation is still useful.

> **Causes of Clubbing**
> Carcinoma bronchus
> Chronic infection
> Fibrosing alveolitus
> Bacterial endocarditis
> Cirrhosis
> Ulcerative collitis
> Crohns

The nails may also reveal other important systemic problems such as psoriatic pitting or renal osteodystrophy. They can also help establish the patient's demands of their hands, are the nails bitten or finely manicured?

Look for callosities (a working man's hand) in contrast to the skin appearance of Sudeks atrophy (dry, shiny and atrophic).

The nicotine stains of a smoker are worthy of comment.

The skin changes of acute infection are an unlikely exam case but a chronic sinus and nail fold infection are possibilities.

Scars can either be surgical or traumatic. The clues that they give are divided into three catergories;

1 Trauma to underlying structures (Nerve, tendon etc.).
2 Previous surgery (Synovectomy / arthrodesis.).
3 Current problems (Scar tethering, neuroma etc.).

To purely state that "there is a scar" is not usually of merit, but to describe an incision as "transverse on the volar surface over the wrist joint" adds descriptive value.

To confidently describe an incision as "Bruner or modified McGregor" (Z-plasty often used in Dupuytren's surgery) may be inviting a difficult follow up question though.

The point is to be able to describe the anatomical position, shape, size, maturity and problems related to a scar rather than the eponymous name given to it.

The Hand and Wrist

Wasting

Note obvious muscle wasting, this can sometimes give the diagnosis.

1. Thenar wasting –   Median nerve palsy (C8)
2. Hypothenar wasting –   Ulnar nerve palsy (T1)
3. Intrinsic wasting –   Ulnar nerve palsy (T1)

It is of course a false demarcation to consider the hand in complete isolation, although the needs of a book demand such things. Always consider the rest of the upper limb, as wasting in the hand may be due to a lesion at a higher level.

Palpation

The site of tenderness must be defined exactly. This is best achieved by breaking up the hand and wrist into specific areas. From localised tenderness, specific tests can then be performed.

Active and passive movements

Normally the next part of the examination would be palpation, however care is always required in the examination of the hand as several conditions can be exquisitely painful.

Remember the golden rule *"Do not hurt the patient"*, by assessing active movement first, a judgement can be made before touching the patient.

Note the range of movement and whether it is painful. The active movement can then be completed as passive movement, again take care not to hurt the patient. Always compare this to the other side.

It is important to use simple clear language when asking the patient to perform these movements and by demonstrating each movement your request may be better understood.

Specific tests of muscles and muscle groups will be considered later. You may have to tailor your examination depending on the movements demonstrated by the patient. Be guided by your findings and the examiner.

Supination and **pronation** are best appreciated with the patient holding their arms against the chest wall with the elbow at 90°. Ask the patient to twist the forearm 'palm up' and then 'palm down'.

Subtle changes in **dorsiflexion** can be seen in the 'prayer position', **palmarflexion** by the reverse of this position. This may be difficult in the rheumatoid patient with elbow and shoulder movement. Simple direct comparison should be made.

Radial and **ulnar wrist deviation** are best demonstrated and then copied by the patient.

Finger and thumb movements again are best demonstrated and then copied by the patient. Perform the following movements in turn:

Finger flexion and extension.
Finger abduction and adduction.
Thumb extension and flexion.
Thumb abduction and adduction.
Opposition.

The Hand and Wrist

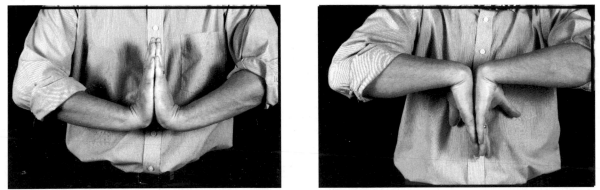

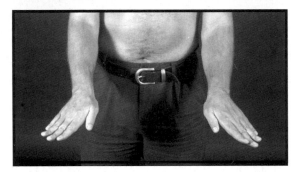

Fig.2 Assess the active range of motion and compare sides for subtle differences.

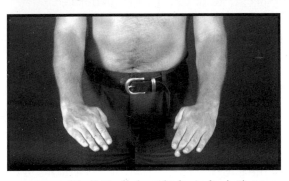

Fig.3 Radial and ulnar deviation

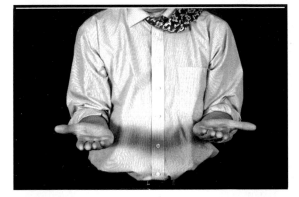

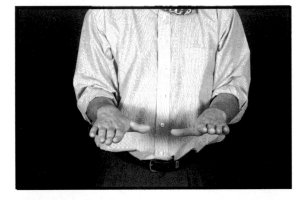

Fig.4 Supination and pronation - Remember to keep the elbows flexed

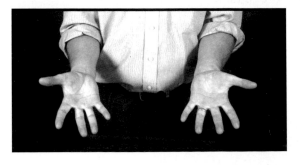

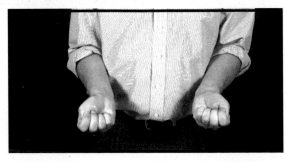

Fig.5 A quick gross assessment of combined joint mobility by open palm and clenched fist.

Special Tests - Specific Muscle Group Testing

The Extrinsic Extensors (the six compartments)

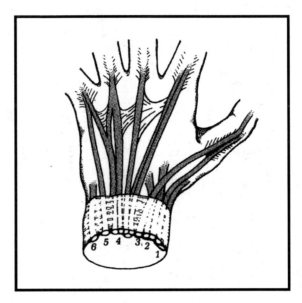

The dorsal compartments of the hand (include a bone with tunnels and description of insertion points). **Remember the mnemonic "221211".**

1. Abductor pollicis longus and extensor pollicis brevis
Abduct the thumb to assess function. (see *Finkelsteins test in deQuervains disease*).

2. Extensor carpi radialis longus and brevis
Test by resisted dorsiflexion of the wrist with the hand clenched. Assess function and palpate tendons.

3. Extensor pollicis longus
Place the hand on the table and lift the thumb on the surface. (Retropulsion)

4. Extensor digitorum communis and extensor indicis proprius
Ask the patient to bring each finger straight with the other fingers bent in a fist.

5. Extensor digiti minimi
As above for the little finger

6. Extensor carpi ulnaris
Dorsiflex and ulnar deviate the hand and feel for the tendon.

Special Tests - Specific Muscle Group Testing

EXTRINSIC EXTENSOR TIGHTNESS

Hold the wrist in neutral. On passively extending the MCPJ the PIPJ should flex. Repeat the test flexing the MCPJs passively, if the PIPJs do not flex then there is extrinsic extensor tightness.

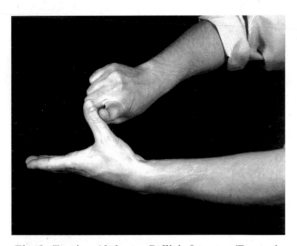

Fig.6   Testing Abductor Pollicis Longus (Posterior interosseous nerve; **C7**, *C8).*

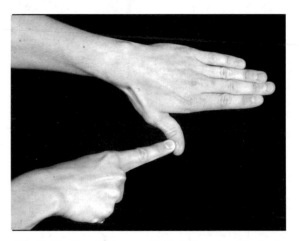

Fig.7   Testing Extensor Pollicis Longus (Posterior interosseous nerve; **C7**, *C8).*

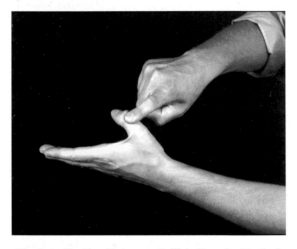

Fig.8   Testing Extensor Pollicis Brevis (Posterior interosseous nerve; **C7**, *C8).*

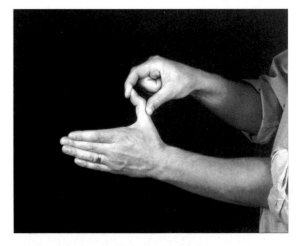

Fig.9   Testing Flexor Pollicis Longus (Anterior interosseous nerve; C7, **C8**).

Special Tests - Specific Muscle Group Testing

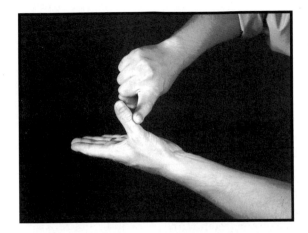

*Fig.10 Testing Abductor Pollicis Brevis (Median nerve; C8, **T1**).*

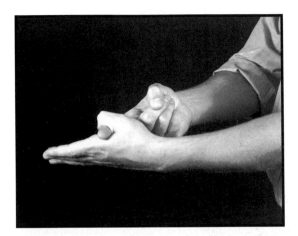

*Fig.11 Testing Opponens Pollicis (Median nerve: C8, **T1**).*

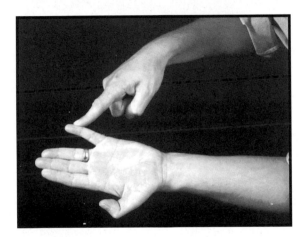

*Fig.12 Testing Abductor Digiti Minimi, (Ulnar Nerve; **C8, T1**) look and feel the muscle belly.*

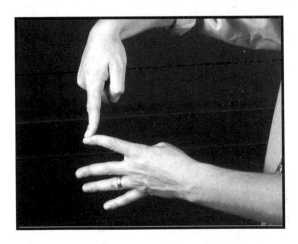

*Fig.13 Testing the First Dorsal Interosseous (Ulnar Nerve; C8, **T1**) again look for and feel the muscle belly.*

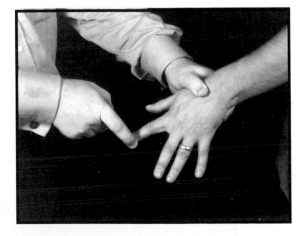

Fig.14 Testing the second Palmer Interosseous. Remember Dorsal ABduct (DAB) and Palmer ADduct (PAD).

Special Tests - Specific Muscle Group Testing

1. Thenar muscles
Together abductor pollicis brevis, opponens pollicis and flexor pollicis brevis can be tested together by touching the little finger to the thumb (the nails need to be parallel). By placing the hand on the dorsum lift the thumb at 90° tests the abductor.

2. Adductor pollicis
'Froments sign' is positive when the distal joint is flexed as a piece of paper is held against the radial border of the hand. *(See Special Tests)*

3. Interossei and lumbricals
The interossei are tested by asking the patient to spread the fingers. Resting the hand flat on the table and hyperextending at the MCPJ tests lumbricals.

4. Hypothenar muscles
The abductor digiti minimi, flexor digiti minimi and opponens digiti minmi are palpated by abducting the little finger away from the others.

INTRINSIC MUSCLE TIGHTNESS
The MCPJ is held in neutral and the PIPJ is passively flexed. This is repeated with the MCPJ in flexion. If the PIPJ cannot be flexed when the MCPJ is extended then there is intrinsic tightness.

Extrinsic Flexors

1. Flexor pollicis longus
Ask the patient to bend the tip of the thumb.

2. Flexor digitorum profundas
Bend the tip of the finger whilst the PIPJ is stabilised

3. Flexor digitorum superficialis
Bend the finger while the other fingers are held in extension.

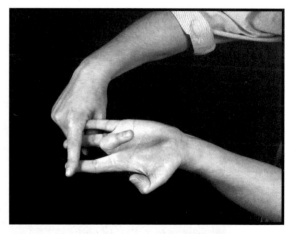

*Fig.15 Testing Flexor Digitorum Superficialis (Median Nerve; C7, **C8**, T1). To eliminate PIPJ movement produced by FDP it is necessary to hold the other fingers extended at the DIPJ.*

4. Flexor carpi ulnaris, flexor carpi radialis and palmaris longus
Holding the wrist in resisted flexion the tendons can be palpated.

Opposition of the little finger and thumb can make the palmaris longus tendon identification easier.

*Fig.16 Testing Flexor Digitorum Profundus (Anterior Interosseous Nerve; C7, **C8**). Note how the PIPJ is blocked.*

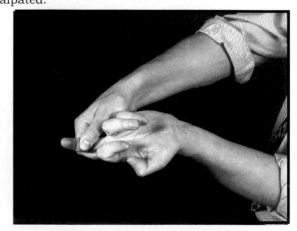

Special Tests - Specific Muscle Group Testing

Instability tests

FINGER AND THUMB LIGAMENT STABILITY TESTS

Technique
The proximal end of the joint is stabilised and valgus, varus, compression and traction stresses are applied.

Clinical implications
The results are compared to the normal side. In the thumb, a valgus angulation of 35° or greater is indicative of significant instability.

References
Heyman P, Gelberman RH, Duncan K, Hipp JA. Injuries of the ulnar collateral ligament of the thumb metacarpophalageal joint.
Clin. Orthop. 1993; 292: 165-71.

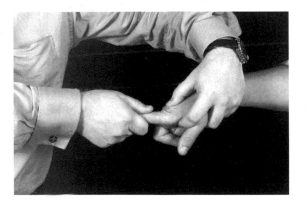

Fig. 17 In a patient with deformity or a history of trauma assessing the stability of joints is vital. Again stability can be quantified as a laxity, soft end point or absent end point etc.

Note the MCPJs should be tested in flexion.

COLLATERAL LIGAMENT TEST

Technique

The PIPJ is held in a neutral position while the DIPJ is passively flexed. The PIPJ is then flexed and DIPJ flexed passively.

Clinical implications
If the DIPJ will not flex with a neutral PIPJ then the collateral ligaments or capsule is tight. If the DIPJ then flexes when the PIPJ is flexed the collaterals are tight but the capsule normal.

Special Tests - Specific Muscle Group Testing

REAGANS TEST (LUNOTRIQUETRAL STABILITY TEST)

Technique

The thumb and second finger of hand grasps the triquetral and the lunate in the other. The lunate is stressed in a dorsal and volar direction.

Clinical implications

Pain and crepitus indicates lunatotriquetral instability

KIRK WATSON TEST (SCAPHOLUNATE STABILITY TEST)

Technique

With the forearm pronated and the hand in ulnar deviation and slight extension the scaphoid is prevented from moving into palmar flexion by the other thumb. The hand is radially deviated and flexed.

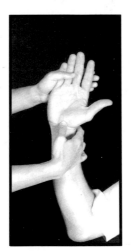

Fig.18 Scaphoid Shift Test. A provaction test of carpal instability in which the scaphoid is stabilised palmarly while the wrist is brought from ulnar to radial deviation. This reproduces the instability feeling and may be associated with a loud "click" if the scaphoid actually subluxes.

Clinical implications

The scaphoid can be felt to sublux over the dorsum of the radius in scapholunate instability.

Modifications

Scaphoid stress test is a modification in which the patient actively radially deviates the hand and the examiner prevents subluxation. If instability is present the scaphoid is forced dorsally.

References

Watson HK, Ashmead D, Maklouf MV. Examination of the scaphoid.
J. Hand Surg. Am. 1988; 70: 1262-68.

Special Tests - Specific Muscle Group Testing

PIANO KEYS TEST

Technique
The distal radio-ulnar joint is stressed.

Clinical implications
Pain and increased mobility indicate distal radioulnar instability.

AXIAL LOADING TEST

Technique
Axial compression is applied to the MCPJ of the thumb.

Clinical implications
Pain or crepitus indicate metacarpo-carpal arthritis.

Modifications
Grind test adds a rotatory movement to localise pathology to the CMCJ.

Tendon and muscle tests

FINKELSTEIN'S TEST

Technique
The patient makes a fist with the thumb inside the fingers. The wrist is pushed into ulnar deviation.

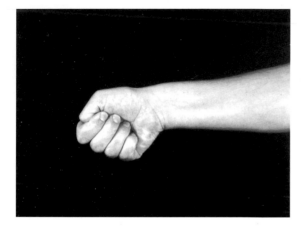

Fig. 19 Finkelstein's Test. Ask the patient to make a fist around their thumb and then Ulnar deviate the wrist. A positive test is recorded if pain results and suggests tenosynovitis of APL and EPB i.e. De Quervain's tenosynovitis.

Clinical implications
Pain and crepitus over abductor pollicis longus is indicative of De Quervians synovitis. This should always be compared to the other side.

References
Finkelstein H. Stenosing tendovagnitis at the radial styloid process.
J. Bone Joint Surg. 1930; 12: 509

Special Tests - Specific Muscle Group Testing

EXTENSOR HOOD TESTS

(Elson's Test) Acute test for Central Slip Disruption.

Technique
The fingers are flexed to 90° over the end of a table and held there. The patient actively extends whilst the examiner palpates the middle phalanx.

Clinical implications
A torn extensor hood results in pressure over the proximal phalanx whilst the distal phalanx rigidly extends.
Negative test when the DIPS remains floppy.

Modifications

Boyes test.
The examiner holds the finger to be examined in slight extension at the PIPJ. A patient with a central slip rupture is unable to flex the DIPJ actively.

References
Elson RA. Rupture of the central slip of the extensor hood of the finger: a test for early diagnosis. *J. Bone Joint Surg. 1986; 68-B: 229-31.*

BUNNEL-LITTLER TEST (INTRINSIC PLUS TEST)

Technique
The MCPJ is held extended and passive flexion of the PIPJ applied. This is repeated with the MCPJ flexed.

Clinical implications
An inability to flex with the joint extended indicates tight capsule or intrinsic muscles. If the joint can be flexed with the MCPJ flexed then the problem is intrinsic tightness.

LINBERGS SIGN

Technique
The patient flexes the thumb on to the hypothenar eminence and actively extends the index finger

Clinical implications
Limited active extension of the index finger is indicative of interconnection between FPL and the index flexors (occurs in 10%)

References
Linburg RM, Cornstock BE. Anomalous tendon slips from flexor pollicis longus to flexor digitorum profundus. *J. Hand Surg. Am. 1979; 4: 79-83.*

Neurological tests

TINEL'S TEST

Technique
Tap over the median nerve at the wrist.

Clinical implications
Parathesia or tingling in the median nerve distribution is indicative of carpal tunnel syndrome.

Remember, Tinel's Test is a sign of nerve regeneration but has been misused in this context to show nerve irritability.

FROMENT'S TEST

Technique
The patient is asked to grasp a piece of paper between the thumb and index finger.

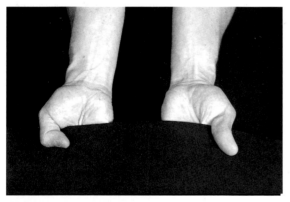

Fig.20 Froment's Test. Ask the patient to hold a piece of card (an X-ray package works well) between the thumb and index finger. Apply traction to the card and compare the posture of both thumbs. Normally the thumb remains flat if it becomes flexed then FPL is being used to assist adductor pollicis suggesting weakness of ulnar function.

Clinical implications
In ulnar paralysis when force is applied to remove the paper the terminal phalanx flexes (as adductor pollicis is paralysed).

Modifications and related tests

Jeanne's sign

Hyperextension of thumb MCPJ during Froment's test indicates adductor pollicis paralysis (ulnar nerve), which acts as an interosseous for the thumb (flexes MCP, extends IPY).

Special Tests - Specific Muscle Group Testing

PHALEN'S TEST

Technique

The wrists are positioned into maximum flexion.

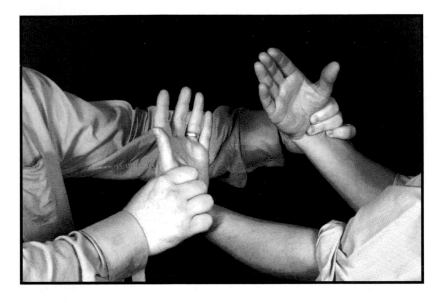

Fig.21 Phalen's Test. Flex both wrists and hold for 60 seconds. Pins and needles, pain etc suggests median nerve entrapment. Some authorities include you holding the patient's hands in this position and using your fingers to increase carpal pressure.

Clinical implications
Tingling in the distribution of the median nerve at 1 minute is indicative of carpal tunnel syndrome.

Modifications and related tests

Reverse Phalen's.
The wrist is extended and direct pressure is applied over the carpal tunnel.

Carpal compression test.
Direct pressure over the carpal tunnel produces median nerve symptoms. This is said to be the most sensitive.

References
Durkan JA. A new diagnostic test for carpal tunnel syndrome.
J. Bone Joint Surg. 1991; 73-A: 535-38

Circulation

ALLEN'S TEST

Technique

The hand is opened and closed and then clenched as tightly as possible. The examiner then presses on both the radial and ulnar arteries and the hand is opened. One is released and the test repeated for the other artery.

Clinical implications

This determines the dominance and patency of the radial and ulnar arteries.

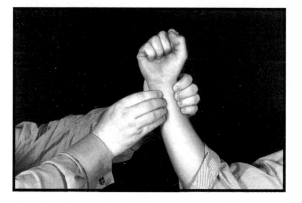 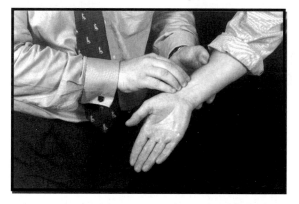

Fig.22 Allen's Test. Ask the patient to elevate their arm, clench the fist a few times, then by digital pressure you occlude both ulnar and radial arteries, lower the arm and release one artery. The hand should rapidly flush, repeat for the other artery. A vital test in the posttraumatic, ITU patient etc to confirm both arteries are patent.

Special Tests - Specific Muscle Group Testing

OTHER TESTS TO ADD:

CUBITAL TUNNEL TEST

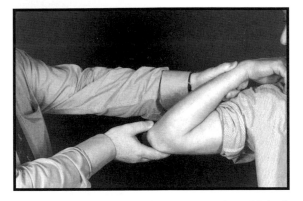

Fig.23 Cubital Tunnel Compression. This is included now as often a part of the hand examination requires a more detailed examination of the ulnar nerve. Flexion of the elbow reproduces the pain or numbness felt by the patient.

TINEL'S TEST

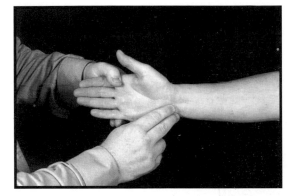

Fig.24 Tinel's Test at Guyon's Canal for ulnar nerve compression at the wrist.

BUNNEL'S "O" SIGN

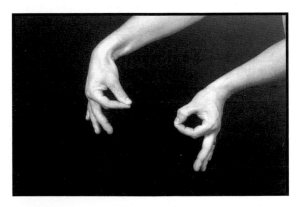

Fig.25 Bunnel's "O" Sign (Kiloh-Nevin Sign). Ask the patient to make an "O" with their thumb and index finger. A patient with Anterior Interosseus Syndrome is weak in both FPL and FDP function and shows hyperextension of the the DIPJ of the index and IPJ of the thumb.

Examination of Hand Swelling

Inspection

Site
Size
Colour
Shape
Scars
Demonstrate effect of active movement

Palpate

Tenderness
Consistency
Edge
Relationship of deep and superficial structures
Mobility

Special Tests

Fluctuations
Pitting
Tinel's test
Crepitus
Sign of emptying
Thrills bruits or pulsatile
Transilluminate
Distal neurovascular status
Palpate regional lymph nodes
Ulcers (edge, floor & base)

Assessment of Hand Function

Precision grips
    tip to tip
    pulp to pulp
    pulp to side

Power grip
    cylinder

    chuck or tripod

    power grasp

    hook

Flat hand

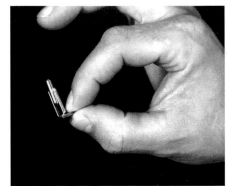

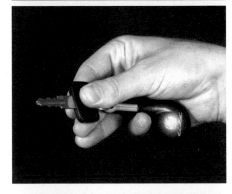

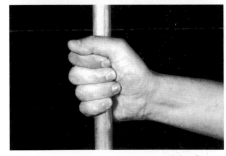

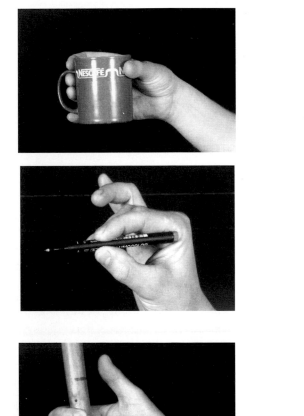

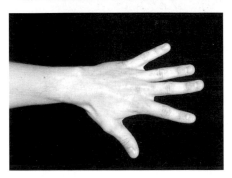

Fig.26 Remember that function is the most important aspect of the examination, even a terribly deformed, burnt out rheumatoid hand may maintain satisfactory function or this may give you a basis to discuss staged procedures and objectives of surgery.

The Arthropathic Hand

Exposure

An initial general description of the hand is often a good opening line i.e. 'generalised symmetrical polyarthropathy affecting mainly the **(MCPs or proximal & distal PIPs)** joints with typical features of **(rheumatoid / psoriatic / degenerative arthropathy)**.

Features are **(e.g ulnar drift, boutonniere deformity, swan neck.....)**.

Screen the neck and shoulders.

Look for skin and nail changes, rheumatoid nodules and bursa on the elbows.

Look specifically for peripheral nerve entrapment.

Specific Joints and Deformities

WRIST AND FOREARM

Look for signs of carpal tunnel syndrome
Head of ulna syndrome
Extensor tendon rupture

FINGERS

Is the deformity fixed or correctable? Check in all positions of adjacent joints and look for intrinsic tightness.
Check for MCPJ dislocation (extensor tendon subluxation, posterior interosseous nerve weakness and perform the tenodesis test).
Look for triggering and tenosynovitis in both flexor and extensor tendons.
Look for tendon rupture, illustrated by a dropped finger but remember, dropped fingers may also be a result of tendon subluxation, joint subluxation or dislocation, posterior interosseus nerve palsy or, in fact a flexor contracture produced by intrinsic tightness.

The Elbow

Mr Stuart Hay MB ChB, FRCS, FRCS(Orth),
Consultant Orthopaedic and Upper Limb Surgeon.

Look

ELBOW EXTENDED   ('PUT YOUR ARMS STRAIGHT')

Deformity	Carrying angle is normally increased in the female with an average of 13° and about 10° in the male. Note any cubitus valgus or varus deformity and start thinking about the causes.
Skin	Old scars, skin grafts, sinuses or erythema.
Contour	
Swelling	Such as that caused by an effusion.
Wasting	Forearm (radial mobile wad and ulnar FDP) Hand (thenar and hypothenar eminence)

ELBOW FLEXED ('SHOW ME YOUR ELBOWS')

Deformity	Prominences and triangle or are the bony land marks concealed by synovial swelling?
Skin	
Contour	
Swelling	Olecranon bursa and RA nodule
Wasting	

MOVE

Extension	**"Straighten your arms"** - normally a female can hyper extend the elbow in comparison to a male but usually no more than 10° from the straight. More than this warrants recording and investigation.
Flexion	**"Bend your arms up"** - the normal range again depends upon several factors in particular depth of soft tissue envelope, about 140° is average.
Rotation	**"Elbows by side bent to 90°"** - then ask patient to face their palms up and then down. Supination is usually slightly more than pronation, normal values respectively of 85° and 80°. It can be difficult to measure this so ensure that you are comparing sides to illustrate any more subtle loss. The extended thumb is a helpful goniometer.

The Elbow

FEEL

Lateral Epicondyle   Tenderness/resisted wrist extension in pronation; resisted middle metacarpal extension.

Radial Head   Tenderness & stability with rotation

Olecranon and Fossa   Bursa. Feel Fossa with elbow unlocked at 30° flexion. Tender Fossa?

Ulnar Nerve   Percussion and Tinel's Test. Stability with flexion/extension - Note position of nerve.

Medial Epicondyle   Tenderness/resisted wrist flexion in supination

Cubital Fossa   Masses/biceps tendon

SPECIAL

Stability   Collateral ligaments
In 30° flexion to unlock Olecranon Fossa
Valgus and varus strain.
Medial and lateral translation.

Pivot Shift

Tennis elbow   can be demonstrated by flexion of the fully pronated forearm and causing pain over the lateral epicondyle by palpation as the elbow is extended.

Golfer's elbow   can be demonstrated by flexion of the supinated forearm and provoking pain by palpation of the medial epicondyle upon extension or during resisted flexion.

Vascular status is important as is neurological examination. One of the most common elective elbow procedures is ulnar nerve transposition.

CLINICAL CASES
Tennis Elbow/Lateral Epicondylitis

Cubital tunnel syndrome

Golfer's Elbow/Medial Epicondylitis

Rheumatoid

Dislocated radial head

Old supracondylar fracture

Radioulnar synostasis

Bony lump

Impingement

The Elbow

Exposure

Again adequate exposure whilst respecting the patients modesty is vital. Any loss of movement in the elbow may be evident when the patient is removing their top. The examination can be performed with the patient sitting or standing.

Inspection

WITH THE ELBOW EXTENDED ('PUT YOUR ARMS STRAIGHT')
Ask the patient to hold the arms out in front of them and look for the following

(a) Deformity
The carrying angle is normally 13° in females and about 10° in the males. Note any cubitus valgus or varus deformity and start thinking about the causes; previous supracondylar-lateral or medial fractures.

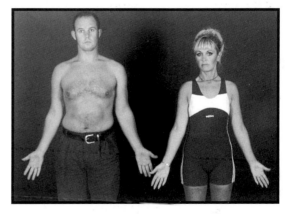

Fig.27 What is the carrying angle of the elbow at rest? Is a Gunstock deformity present from an old mal-united supracondylar fracture?

(b) Skin
Look for old scars, skin grafts, sinuses or erythema. Paper-like skin of Ehlers -Danlos Syndrome.

(c) Contour and Swelling
The swelling of an effusion or synovitis may be visible around the joint. Look at the soft spot of the infra-condylar recess.

(d) Wasting
Look at the forearm. Wasting in the radial mobile wad and ulnar FDP may indicate nerve injury higher up. In the hand, wasting of the thenar or hypothenar eminences may give you further clues.

The Elbow

ELBOW FLEXED ('SHOW ME YOUR ELBOWS')

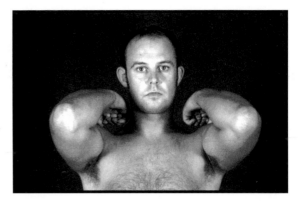

Fig.28 Show me your elbows! An old scar from ORIF of an olecranon fracture or olecranon bursitis may be more obvious in this position.

(a) Deformity

Comment on any noticeable prominences and any disruption in the normal 'elbow triangle'. Synovial swelling can conceal bony landmarks. Look at the infra-condylar recess.

(b) Skin

Again describe any scars, sinuses or skin changes.

(c) Contour and Swelling

An olecranon bursa or rheumatoid nodule may be present. The latter may point you to comment on the typical changes of a rheumatoid hand.

(d) Wasting

Note any wasting in the forearm and upper arm.

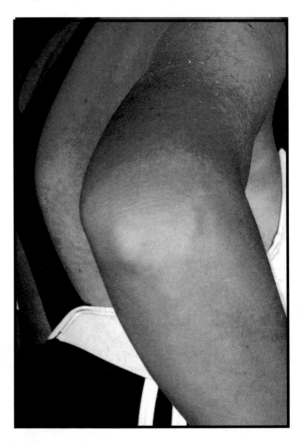

Fig.29 Look at the elbow itself. Do the three bony landmarks of medial, lateral epicondyle and olecranon form an even triangle in flexion? Is there normal muscle bulk?

The Elbow

Movement

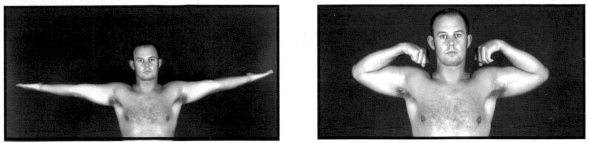

Fig.30 Flexion and extension. Always compare sides. The forearm can be used as a useful goniometer.

Movement is best appreciated from the front. Active movement can be followed by passive completion of movement and the range noted. Comparison with the normal side is very helpful. Abduction of shoulders with supination of forearm for flexion and extension allows the forearm to act as a goniometer.

EXTENSION

"Straighten your arms" - normally a female can hyper extend the elbow in comparison to a male but usually no more than 10°, more than this warrants a comment and further investigation locally and overall (maybe a case of general hyperlaxity).

FLEXION

"Bend your arms up" - the normal range depends upon several factors in particular depth of soft tissue envelope, about 140° is average.

ROTATION

With the elbows by side and bent to 90° ask patient to face their palms up and then down (demonstrating this may be more helpful and make for a smoother examination). Supination is usually slightly more than pronation, 85° compared to 80°. It can be difficult to measure this so ensure that you are comparing sides to illustrate any more subtle loss. The extended thumb is a useful goniometer.

Fig.31 Pronation and supination deficits can be compensated for by glenohumeral motion. Hold the elbow at 90° to limit this effect. A pencil held in the hand can act as a useful prop to demonstrate subtle differences.

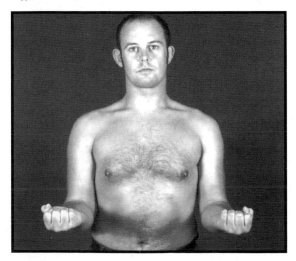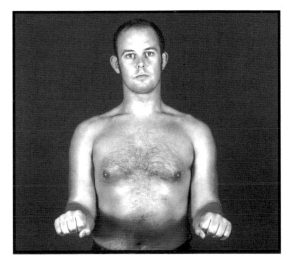

The Elbow

Palpation

As with all joints a systematic approach will make the overall examination easier and will stop you forgetting any parts. This can be achieved by starting laterally and "circumnavigating" the joint.

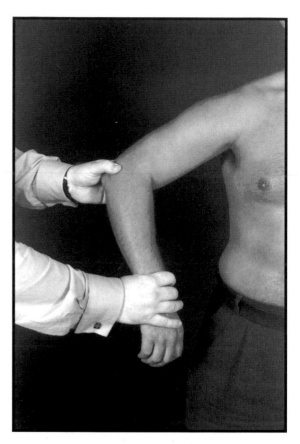

(a) Lateral Epicondyle
Elicit any localised tenderness, consider tennis elbow and perform appropriate tests.

(b) Radial Head
Tenderness particularly on forearm rotation may indicate radial head pathology. Test the stability of the joint and any crepitus.

Fig. 32 Palpation should be performed in a logical and organised manner. "Circumnavigate" the elbow, starting at the lateral epicondyle and finishing in the antecubital fossa. Elicit tenderness, crepitation and loose bodies.

(c) Olecranon and Fossa
Feel for an olecranon bursa, describe it as you would any swelling and think of a differential diagnosis. Tenderness in fossa with posterior impingement.

(d) Ulnar Nerve
Percussion to elicit any sensitivity as with Tinel's Test. Flex and extend the elbow, feeling the nerve and comment on instability. Think of the elbow with cubitus valgus and a tardy ulna nerve.

(e) Medial Epicondyle
Elicit any localised tenderness, consider Golfers Elbow and perform appropriate tests.

(f) Antecubital Fossa
Feel for any masses and palpate the biceps tendon. Active flexion and supination against resistance will reveal a ruptured biceps tendon. Occasional anterior tenderness with anterior impingement.

Finally feel distal pulses and assess the neurological status.

The Elbow

Special Tests

LIGAMENTOUS TESTS

INSTABILITY TEST

Technique

The lateral structures are tested with the elbow held at 30° (advised to be undertaken with the humerus internally rotated. The medial structures are tested in the opposite direction and rotation.)

Clinical implications

Opening with a poor end-point is indicative of instability.

PIVOT SHIFT TEST

Technique

The examiner stands above the head of the supine patient. The examiner supports the distal humerus with one hand while the other supinates the forearm, while applying axial compression and a valgus force. The elbow is then flexed and extended. Apprehension with or without subluxation is felt with the extending elbow, this reduces in flexion.

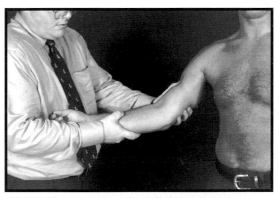

Fig.33 The lateral and medial support structures of the elbow are tested by valgus varus testing. It is important to hold the elbow at 30°, this unlocks the mechanical support of the olecranon and trochlear groove.

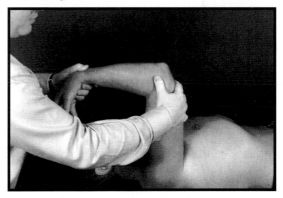

Fig.34 The Pivot Shift Test. With the patient supine and the elbow and shoulder flexed to 90°, stand behind the patient, supinate their forearm, axial compression, valgus strain and then flex and extend their elbow.

The Elbow

LATERAL EPICONDYLITIS
(TENNIS ELBOW)

Technique
Stabilise the elbow by resting the thumb on the lateral epicondyle. The patient makes a fist, pronates the forearm, radially deviates and flexes the wrist.

Clinical implications
Pain is a sign of Tennis Elbow.

Modifications and related tests

Mills' modification is simply the application of this movement by the examiner by resisted wrist extension.

Middle finger test. Resisted extension of the index finger induces the pain in the lateral epicondyle.

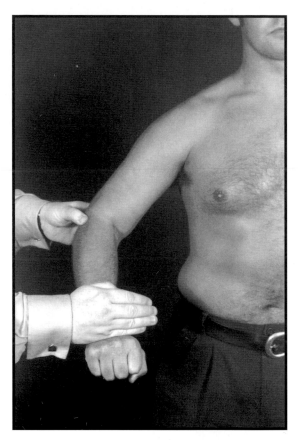

Fig.35 Cozen's Test (Mills' modifications) For lateral epicondylitis, stabilise the elbow by resting a thumb on the lateral epicondyle, ask the patient to bend their elbow while extending the wrist with a clenched fist. Resist this wrist extension and pain will be felt around the lateral epicondyle.

The Elbow

MEDIAL EPICONDYLITIS (GOLFER'S ELBOW)

Technique

The medial epicondyle is palpated and forearm is supinated and wrist extended. Resisted wrist flexion when combined with palpation may also produce a positive response.

Clinical implications

Pain is indicative of golfer's elbow.

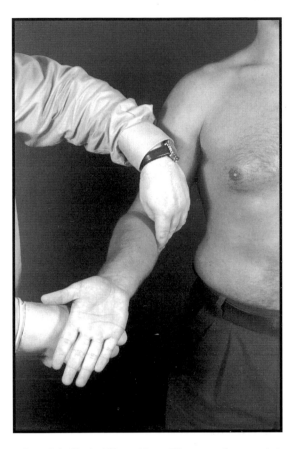

Fig.36 Golfer's Elbow Test. The examiner resists the extension of the patient's elbow by pressure against the back of their supinated, extended hand.

The Elbow

NEUROLOGICAL TESTS

ULNAR NERVE DYSFUNCTION

Technique

A Tinel's sign can be elicted over the elbow behind the medial epicondyle.

Clinical implications

This is indicative of ulnar neuropathy

Modifications and related tests

Elbow " Phalen's type" test. The elbows are maximally flexed and wrists extended and this position held for 5 minutes. Ulnar nerve compression results in neurological changes in the distribution of the nerve.

RADIAL TUNNEL SYNDROME

Technique

Tapping over the medial (supinator) tunnel in the line of the deep branch of the radial nerve may reproduce symptoms suggestive of Radial Tunnel Syndrome, with pain radiating into the dorsal-lateral forearm. Pain only a problem without motor or sensory dysfunction.

IMPINGEMENT

Forced extension and forced flexion should not be painful to perform. Posterior pain with extension is suggestive of posterior impingement while anterior pain in fored flexion is suggestive of anterior impingement (between the coronoid tip and the coronoid fossa). Likewise, symptoms may be elicited by deep palpation in the olecranon and antecubital fossa respectively.

The Shoulder

Mr Richard M F Hill FRCS Ed.
Specialist Registrar, Trauma and Orthopaedics.

Mr Cormac Kelly FRCS,FRCS(Orth).
Consultant Orthopaedic and Upper Limb Surgeon.

Mr Joby John MRCS
Specialist Registrar

EXPOSURE

To waist, respect the modesty of patient.
Watch them undress and comment on it as
well as any aids.

INSPECTION

Start anteriorly, work laterally and end
posteriorly commenting on each category.

Deformity & Contours	Head and neck SCJ Clavicle ACJ Shoulder height Arm position Scapular symmetry (height and winging) Rest of Body	
Skin	Scars.	
Wasting	Pectoral Deltoid Biceps (may require resisted elbow flexion) Trapezius Supraspinatus Infraspinatus	

Shoulder Pathology	
Young	-Instability, bursitis
Middle age	-Frozen shoulder -Calcific tendinitis -Impingement
Old	-Cuff tear -Osteoarthritis

PALPATION

Start anteriorly, work laterally and end posteriorly in a systematic order.
State intention to examine neck (Know Spurlings sign, see Figure 1).

Joints & bony skeleton	SCJ Clavicle ACJ (ACJ pain is worse with Scarf test) Anterior humeral head and Acromion Coracoid (Tenderness common and non specific) Humeral head and axillary lymph nodes Lateral acromion and deltoid origin Scapular spine Medial boarder of scapula Superior and inferior fossa for loss of muscle bulk.
Palpable swellings	SCJ Subluxation / dislocation Clavicular fracture / non-union ACJ Dislocation Ganglion and osteophytes of ACJ Subacromial bursa Anterior head dislocation Prominent coracoid (Consider posterior dislocation / subluxation)

The Shoulder

MOVEMENT

From behind the patient.

Forward flexion in plane of scapula (thumb down arm forward)

Abduction (thumb up palms forwards)

From the side of the patient

Extension
Functional Internal rotation (measure at the level of mid-palm)
External rotation (at side and at 90 deg abduction)
Adduction

POWER

Trapezius	Shoulder shrug
Rhomboids	Elbow extension against resistance
Serratus Anterior	Push off wall
Latissimus dorsi	Resisted adduction
Deltoid (3 parts)	Abduction at 90 degrees
Pectoralis Major	Resisted adduction
Supraspinatus	Thumb down in 30 deg forward flexion
Infraspinatus & Teres minor	Resist external rotation arm at side
Subscapularis	Gerber's and Napoleon tests

IMPINGEMENT TESTS
Neer's impingement sign.
Neer's impingement injection test.
Hawkins-Kennedy test.

BICEPS PROVOCATION TESTS

Speed's test
Yergason's test

INSTABILITY TESTS

Patient sitting initially arm on the lap. Ask about voluntary component.

Inferior	Sulcus sign
Anterior	Load and shift test
	Apprehension test
	Jobes relocation test

Patient lying down.

Posterior	Posterior apprehension test
	Norwood stress test

Labral tests

Clunk Test
SLAP Test

THORACIC OUTLET SYNDROME
Adson's Test
Wright's Test
Roos Test

The Shoulder

The shoulder girdle consists of three bones, four joints and is surrounded by a musculotendinous cuff. The shoulder is the most mobile joint in the body and relies on soft tissues for stability. As a result concise yet methodical approach is required if salient points are not to be missed. Always compare with the asymptomatic normal side. It is easier to perform the whole examination with the patient standing but in a frail patient it is not unreasonable to allow them to sit throughout inspection and palpation. Certain tests especially in instability require the patient to be supine. Also remember that certain conditions occur commonly at different ages (See table 1).

Young	- Instability, bursitis
Middle age	- Frozen shoulder - Calcific tendinitis - Impingement
Old	- Cuff tear - Osteoarthritis

Table 1

NECK EXAMINATION

Always mention your eagerness to examine the neck, as shoulder pain can be referred from the cervical spine e.g. cervical root stenosis. A brief examination of the active and passive range of movement only takes a minute. Are neck movement's painful? **Spurling's sign** is indicative of cervical root tension. Reproduction of the patient's pain with ipsilateral rotation and flexion is a positive result (Figure 1).

Reference:
Spurling RG, Scoville WB. Lateral rupture of the cervical intervertebral discs:
A common cause of shoulder and arm pain.
Surg gynecol Obstet 1944;78: 350-8.

Fig.1.

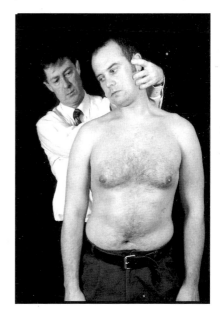

EXPOSURE

Ask the patient to undress to the waist but always respect the patient's modesty. Close observation will provide some idea of the degree of pain and the patient's functional disability. Make a comment on this, even if normal and mention the use of any aids. Remember the requirement for walking sticks or a wheelchair increases the chance of rotator cuff disease and also influences rehabilitation.

The Shoulder

INSPECTION

Walk around the patient looking at the front, side and posterior aspect of the shoulder. This is best undertaken in a logical pattern as described below. Again it is useful to communicate your findings at each stage.

FROM THE FRONT & SIDE
DEFORMITY & CONTOUR

Comment on any obvious neck or upper thoracic deformity. It may be a source of referred shoulder pain. Some women with large breasts get poor scapular position leading to impingement. The shoulder heights and supraclavicular fossa should be compared and asymmetry noted. From the midline note any sternoclavicular joint prominence (e.g. subluxation, tumour, infection or osteophytes). Follow along the clavicle noting any deformity (suggestive of an old fracture) to the acromio-clavicular joint. Remember prominance of the ACJ may be normal and ganglions, effusion and synovitis are common causes of swellings. Diffuse swelling of the sub-acromial bursa can be subtle and seen antero-lateral to the acromion.

SKIN & SCARS

Comment on scars from previous surgery or accidents with close inspection of the neck as well. A scar in the posterior triangle should alert you to the possibility of iatrogenic trapezius palsy. Always look carefully for the scars of arthroscopy portals (posterior, lateral and anterior).

WASTING

Gross pectoral wasting can be seen from the front. This has both congenital and acquired causes. Diffuse deltoid wasting commonly is seen in patients with long term stiffness. Anterior deltoid wasting should alert you to the possibility of axillary nerve palsy. This sometimes occurs after shoulder dislocation or previous surgery. Deltoid detachment to varying degrees can be seen after open shoulder surgery. Long-head of biceps rupture is usually obvious but sometimes requires resisted elbow flexion with forearm supination.

The Shoulder

FROM BEHIND AND ABOVE

DEFORMITY & CONTOUR

Look at the size, shape and relative height of the scapula. (See table 2). Winging of the scapula can be specifically tested for by asking the patient to press both arms against the wall (Figure 2 & 3). Squaring off of the shoulder due to Deltoid wasting is most notable from behind

Abnormal scapular
Sprengel shoulder
(small & high)
Klippel - Feil syndrome (webbed neck)
Winged scapular
Trapezius or Serratus anterior palsy

Table 2

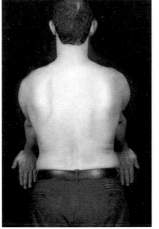

Fig.2

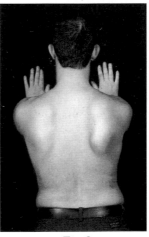

Fig.3

SKIN & SCARS

Again arthroscopy portals must be sought. Posterior surgical scars are rare and may indicate previous fracture fixation or rarely posterior stabilisation.

WASTING

Trapezius and deltoid wasting; in particular the posterior and middle fibres, are best visualised from behind. You must comment on rotator cuff wasting and close inspection of the supra-scapular and infra-scapular are vital. Assessment is aided by comparing the prominence of the scapular spines and it is appropriate to gently palpate each fossa for bulk comparing both sides. Wasting is usually due to rotator cuff tears but do not forget other pathologies such as suprascapular nerve compression and brachial plexus dysfunction.

The Shoulder

PALPATION

Before palpation ask the patient to point to any painful areas and rate them according to severity. Pain from the acromio-clavicular joint (ACJ is easily localised by the patient with one finger (figure 4) whilst sub-acromial pain is poorly localised to the anterior lateral area of the shoulder (figure 5).

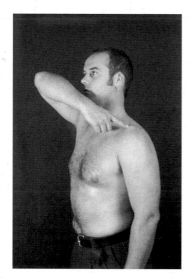

Fig.4

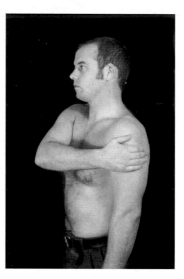

Fig.5

The sternoclavicular joint is palpated standing from the side using the right hand on the right shoulder and vice versa. Follow the clavicle to the acromio-clavicular joint commenting on any tenderness. Localised ACJ pain that is exacerbated with passive adduction of the arm across the chest is considered a positive Scarf test.
Move your fingers anterior and lateral to the acromion and palpate for Subacromial tenderness and swelling both in neutral and in slight extension. It is the authors' belief that the presence and extent of rotator cuff tears cannot reliably be elicited by palpation. Coracoid tenderness is often non-specific and it is difficult to elicit biceps tendon tenderness. The upper humeral shaft and head can be palpated via the axilla with the arm passively abducted. Other axillary swellings can also appreciated at this stage. Painless axillary nodes may indicate neighbouring malignancy.

MOVEMENT

Movements are best appreciated from behind with the patient standing in front of a mirror. If a full-length mirror is not available explain this is what you would normally do. It allows you to be able to observe facial expression whilst observing (still) from the back. Comment on any trick movements patients use during movement. Examine each movement actively and then complete the arc passively. Beware of causing undue pain as this may limit the usefulness of further examination. Examining the asymptomatic or normal side first gives an indication of the normal range of movement. Always consider simultaneous bilateral movements especially forward flexion and abduction. A goniometer always impresses and provides a more accurate assessment of range of movement.

The Shoulder

FORWARD FLEXION occurs in the plane of the scapula; 30 degrees lateral to the coronal plane (Figure 6). Always note and comment on the scapular rhythm. The normal range is 0 to 160-180 degrees and is a combination of gleno-humeral and scapulo-thoracic components with an average ratio of 2:1. In the 1st 25 degrees it is 4:1 and then 5:4 over 25 - 180 degrees of flexion.

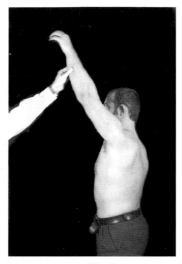

Fig.6

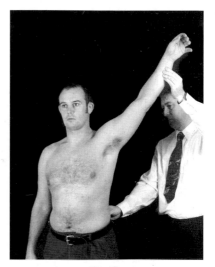

Fig.7

ABDUCTION is best assessed by asking the patient to lift both arms out sideways simultaneously with palms facing forwards (Figure 7). Again comment on the rhythm and the total active and passive movement. Normal range of movement is 0 to 170° (0-90° gleno-humeral >90° scapulothoracic). It is important to appreciate each specific component. If the gleno-humeral joint is stiff (osteoarthritis, frozen shoulder) then all movement will occur in the scapulo-thoracic joint. By fixing the position of the scapula with one hand and gently abducting the humerus the true portion of each joint motion can be confirmed.

The painful arc is seen when the mid arc of forward flexion and abduction is painful. It indicates pain from the sub-acromial bursa often seen in impingement and rotator cuff tears. A high painful arc is often but not exclusively seen in acromioclavicular joint osteoarthritis. Difficulty in initiating abduction can indicate a rotator cuff lesion.

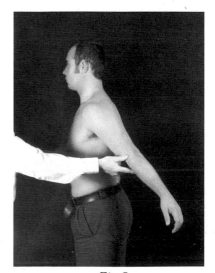

EXTENSION Is best viewed from the side. Ask the patient to lift their arm backwards. The normal range is 0 to 60°. (Figure 8).

Fig.8

ADDUCTION this best viewed from the front by asking the patient to bring their arm across the chest. The normal range is 0 to 50°. Loss of adduction is commonly seen in frozen shoulder (Figure 9). Painful passive adduction (Scarf test) often exaggerates the pain of ACJ pathology.

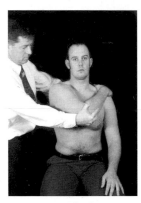

Fig.9

EXTERNAL ROTATION needs to be tested in adduction and abduction to enable evaluation of which structures are tight if any. First fix the elbow to the chest wall and ask the patient to externally rotate their forearm. Then abduct the arm to ninety degrees and repeat the manoeuvre. It is best to evaluate the normal side first and to follow each active with passive testing. The normal range is variable 0 to 70°. (Figure 10 & 11). Females usually have greater movement due to greater joint laxity. Testing external rotation of the patient in abduction may produce apprehension, which may indicate anterior instability (vide infra).

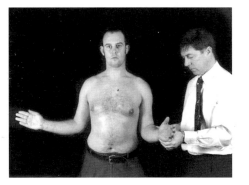

Fig.10

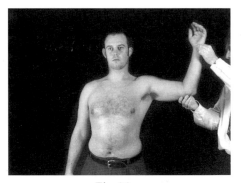

Fig.11

FUNCTIONAL INTERNAL ROTATION is a combination of extension and humeral internal rotation. It is measured by asking the patient to put their hand up their back. Measure the height of the mid-palm according to the vertebral level i.e. lateral thigh, buttock, sacro-iliac joint, S1, L5, and L4 etc. Normality is variable but most patients can reach to T6, T7 area (Figure 12). True internal rotation is evaluated with arm at the side with the elbow extended. Place your fingers and thumb on the medial and lateral condyles of the humerus and internally rotate the arm. Estimate the degree of internal rotation and compare with the other side.

Fig.12

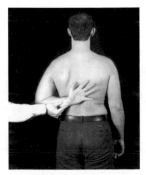

The Shoulder

MUSCLE TESTING

It is important to assess the integrity and power of specific muscle groups, especially the muscles of the rotator cuff. Describe which muscle is being tested, its power and comment upon whether testing is painful. Start with the posterior muscles and move round to the anterior muscles and end with the biceps and other arm muscles if clinically indicated.

THE POSTERIOR MUSCLES

Trapezius is palpated whilst the patient holds the shoulders shrugged. Resisting this motion tests power. Weakness results in winging of the scapula with it classically being displaced downwards and outwards, with the upper portion of the scapula moving away from the midline.

Rhomboids activity can be assessed by resisting extension of the shoulder. Winging of the scapula is seen with weakness.

Serratus anterior is tested by asking the patient to lean against the wall with both hands, winging of the scapula again becomes apparent with weakness. Here the scapula classically moves upwards and inwards, with inferior angle moving towards the spinous processes.

Latissmus dorsi extends, internally rotates and is a powerful adductor of the arm. Abducting the arm to 90 degrees and resisting adduction tests it and the muscle can be easily felt below the posterior axillary fold.

THE ANTERIOR MUSCLES

The deltoid is critical for good shoulder function. It has three parts, the anterior, middle and posterior heads. One or all may be dysfunctional due to injury or denervation. Anterior deltoid wasting is usually due to iatrogenic nerve injury or inadequate reattachment after rotator cuff surgery. Global deltoid dysfunction is seen after fractures and dislocations of the glenohumeral joint due to injury of the axillary nerve.

Ask the patient to hold the arm in 90 degrees of abduction. The three heads of deltoid should be palpable

The Shoulder - Special Tests

Pectoralis major is tested by palpation with resisted adduction of the arm.

Biceps rupture is common and is tested by resisted flexion. Any rupture can then be visualised and palpated.

Supraspinatus is best tested bilaterally and simultaneously. Place the patient's arms in 30-60° flexion in the scapular plane with thumbs turned downwards and ask them to resist downward pressure (Figure13). It is the authors opinion that supraspinatus is a major contributor to the initiation of flexion and abduction.

Infraspinatus & teres minor are tested by resisted external rotation with the elbow flexed to 90° to the chest wall (Figure 14).

Subscapularis is best evaluated by Gerbers lift-off test (Figure 15). Ask the patient to place the back of their hand into the small of their back. The ability to lift the hand from the back indicates an intact subscapularis. Power is evaluated in the usual way vide infra. Pain or stiffness can prevent some patients placing their hand into the small of the back in which case the **Napoleon** sign is used. Ask the patient to place their palm on the abdomen and bring their elbow forward. Patients with complete subscapularis rupture are unable to perform this manoeuvre (Figure16). Remember that subscapularis is rarely ruptured in isolation.

Gerber's lift-off test was based on the observation that weakness of internal rotation is most easily demonstrated at the limit of muscles amplitude; when the arm is extended and internally rotated. A positive test in combination with increased passive external rotation indicates complete subscapularis rupture.

Reference

Gerber C, Krushell RJ. Isolated ruptures of the tendon of the subscapularis muscle. J. Bone Joint Surg. 1991, 73-B: 389-94

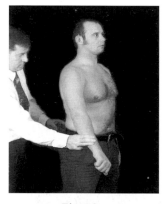

Fig. 13

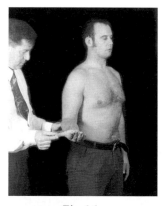

Fig. 14

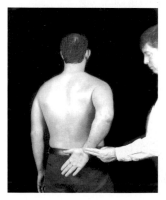

Fig. 15

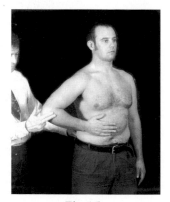

Fig.16

The Shoulder - Special Tests

LAG SIGNS

Lag signs are positive in severe weakness or muscle disruption. This sign is often used for supraspinatus and infraspinatus. When testing supraspinatus the patient is asked to hold the position of forward flexion of 90 degrees. A positive sign is when the arm gradually drops as the secondary recruited muscles fatigue. For infraspinatus the patient is asked to keep the forearm in full external rotation with the elbow flexed to 90 degrees and held in against the chest wall. Severe weakness is identified if the forearm drifts towards neutral rotation.

SPECIAL TESTS

There are numerous specialist tests to detect abnormalities in the shoulder. The authors recommend the routine use of a limited number of tests as described below.

IMPINGEMENT TESTS

With the patient standing, impingement is assessed using **Neer's impingement sign** and **test (injection test)** and **Hawkin's Kennedy test.**

NEER'S IMPINGEMENT SIGN & TEST

Neer's impingement sign is carried out by passively elevating the patient's arm in the scapular plane. This jams the greater tuberosity against the anteroinferior of the acromion and coracoacromial ligament. A positive test results in pain often reflected in the patient's facial expression. (Figure 17). If a positive result is identified, inform the examiner that you would like to proceed to Neer's impingement test. Local anaesthetic is injected into the sub-acromial space. Ten minutes later the procedure is repeated. If the patient's pain is alleviated it is recorded as a positive result.

Three stages of impingement are described by Neer; stage I, oedema and haemorrhage of the tendons; stage II, fibrosis and tendinitis; stage III, bony spurs and tendon ruptures.

Reference
Neer CS, Welsh RP. The shoulder in sports. Orthop. Clin. North Am. 1977, 8: 3: 583-9

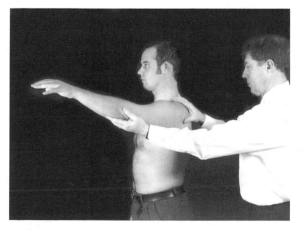

Fig. 17

The Shoulder - Special Tests

HAWKIN'S KENNEDY TEST.

The arm is passively forward flexed to 90° and then internally rotated. This movement forces the supraspinatus tendon against the anterior surface of coracoacromial ligament and coracoid process. Reproduction of the patient's pain is a positive test and is indicative of supraspinatus pathology. (Figure 18).

Reference
Hawkins RJ, Kennedy JC. Impingement syndrome in atheletes. Am. J. Sports Med. 1980; 8: 151-63

BICEPS PROVOCATION TESTS

Bicipital pathology is assessed by **Speed's** and **Yergason's test**

SPEED'S TEST

Increased anterior shoulder pain is experienced with resisted forward elevation of the arm at 90 degrees (Figure 19). Increased pain in the bicipital grooves indicates bicipital tendinitis. This test is not considered very specific and can be positive with suraspinatus pathology.

Reference
Rockwood CA. Subluxations and dislocations about the shoulder. In Rockwood CA & Green DP (eds): The Shoulder. Philadelphia, Lippincott . 1984

YERGASON'S TEST

The elbow is flexed to 90° and the forearm is pronated. Ask the patient to supinate and try and resist this movement (Figure 20). Pain in the shoulder with resisted supination can indicate tendinitis or rupture of the long head of biceps.

Reference
Yergason RM. Supination sign. J. Bone Joint Surg. 1931; 13: 160

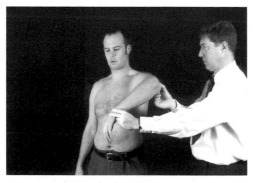

Fig.18

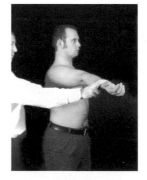

Fig.19

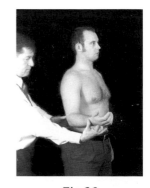

Fig.20

The Shoulder - Special Tests

INSTABILITY TESTS

Instability should be evaluated in both the sitting and lying positions. Before undertaking instability tests always inform the examiner of what you are about to do. Whilst the patient is positioning himself or herself it is always worth asking the patient if they feel their shoulder feels unstable and in what position. The history and/or previous x-rays may help in deciding on the direction of dislocations. Anterio-inferior subluxation and dislocation are by far the most common injury. Ask if they are able to dislocate and relocate their own shoulder at will. This will help decide on any component of voluntary dislocation. The purpose of the examination is to assess joint laxity, pain and apprehension.

INFERIOR INSTABILITY

The **sulcus sign** assesses inferior laxity (Figure 21). With the patient standing fix the scapula between the thumb and forefinger over the anterior acromion and scapula spine. Then provide traction in line with the humerus with the arm in neutral rotation and 20-50 degrees of abduction. A hollowing below the acromion is positive and can be graded by measuring the distance between the inferior aspect of the acromion and the humeral head. Grade I is 0-1, grade II is 1-2 and grade III is >2cm.

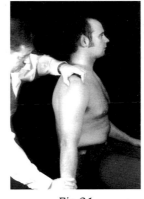

Fig.21

ANTERIO-INFERIOR INSTABILITY

Anterior instability is evaluated with Load shift test and apprehension test. If the patient shows evidence of anterior-inferior instability move on to Jobe's relocation test in the supine position. The degree of translation is measured according to Hawkins and Mohtadi three-grade system (See table 3.)

Table 3.

Grading of anterior draw test	
0	<25% normal
1	Between 25%-50%
2	Between 50%-100%
3	Can be dislocated.
N.B in posterior test 50% is normal.	

The Shoulder - Special Tests

Load Shift Test

The patient sits comfortably with the palm of their hands resting on their thighs. Stand behind the patient stabilising the scapula. This is carried out using the opposite hand to the side of the shoulder. Place your index finger on the coracoid and thumb on the scapula. With your other hand hold the head of humerus with the thumb over the posterior aspect wrapping the fingers anteriorly. Gently push the humerus forwards carrying out the load part of the test, relocating the humeral head into the centre of the glenoid. The examiner then pushes the head forward noting the degree of translation. This is the shift portion of the test. Translation of up to 25% of the diameter of the head is normal (Figure 22a & b). Comparison between the normal and affected shoulder should be made and is more important than any single value. Comparison between the amount and the ease of translation should be made.

A 'clunk' occurring when the test is being performed may indicate a labral tear or Bankart lesion. Further **Labral tests** can be performed to help confirm the clinical diagnosis (Vide infra)

Reference
Hawkins RJ, Mohtadi NG. Clinical evaluation of shoulder instability. Clin. J. Sports Med. 1991; 1: 59-64.

Apprehension Test

With the patient still sitting it is possible to carry out the apprehension test. This test needs to be carried out slowly and with care since it is possible to dislocate the humeral head with this manoeuvre. Abduct the arm to 90 degrees and then slowly externally rotate the arm (Figure 23). Pay close attention to the patients face. A positive test is identified with by a look or feeling of apprehension and the patient's resistance to further external rotation. The patient may also state that this reproduces the discomfort that they usually experience. Note the degree of external rotation at which their apprehension occurred. The same test but with the patient in the supine position is sometimes known as the Crank test. A positive test should be followed by **Jobe's** relocation test.

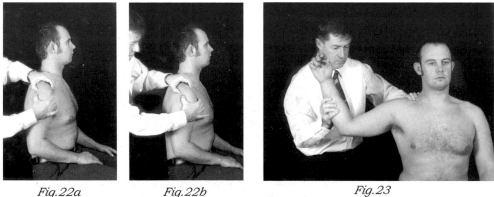

Fig.22a   *Fig.22b*   *Fig.23*

The Shoulder - Special Tests

Relocation (Jobe's) Test

In the supine position the patients arm is once again abducted to 90 degrees and external rotation carried out. Once the point of apprehension is reached place the palm of the hand on the anterior aspect of the humerus and apply a posterior stress. If positive the patient will lose their apprehension or pain and this allows further external rotation (Figure 24). Should the relocation test increase the degree of pain or discomfort consider posterior instability, impingement or arthritis as the underlying pathology.

POSTERIOR-INFERIOR INSTABILITY

Posterio-inferior instability is rare compared to anterior-inferior instability. It is best tested in the supine position and common tests include **Posterior apprehension** and **Norwood stress tests**. Note that 50% posterior translation can be achieved in normal individuals.

Posterior apprehension or stress test

Hold the patient's left arm at the wrist with your right hand. Flex the shoulder to 90 degrees in the scapular plane with the elbow flexed to 90 degrees. Then apply an axial force to the shoulder. Laying your right forearm along the patient's forearm can easily control this. Whilst applying the axial load gently adduct and medially rotate the forearm. A positive result is indicated by pain or apprehension with the patient resisting further movement. Pagnani and Warren reported that pain is more likely than apprehension and that the test is negative in multidirectional instability.

Reference

Pollack RG, Bigliani LU. Recurrent posterior shoulder instability: diagnosis and treatment. Clin. Orthop. 1993; 291:85-96.

Pagnani MJ and Warren RF: Multidirectional instability in the athlete. In Pettrone FA (ed): Athletic Injuries of the Shoulder. New York, McGraw-Hill ., 1995

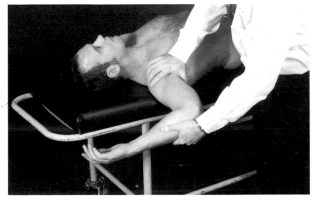

Fig.24

The Shoulder - Special Tests

Norwood Stress test

With patient supine the shoulder is placed in a position of 90 degrees of abduction and neutral rotation. Stabilise the scapula and palpate the posterior aspect of the humeral head with the other hand. Then adduct the arm across the chest feeling for posterior head subluxation (Figure 25a & b). Care should be taken as this test can cause subluxation or dislocation without apprehension. Translation of more than 50% of the humeral head indicates a positive test.

Reference
Norwood LA, Terry GC. Shoulder posterior subluxation. Am. J. Sports Med. 1984; 12: 25-30

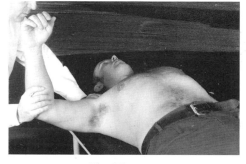
Fig.25a

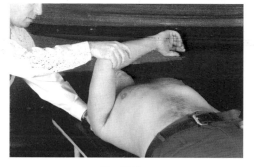
Fig.25b

LABRAL TESTS

The aims of labral tests are to try and identify a Bankart labral injury. The tests are non-specific, numerous and varied. The clunk test is perhaps the most often performed.

CLUNK TEST

With the patient supine with one hand is placed on the posterior aspect of the shoulder whilst the other holds the humerus above the elbow. The arm is fully abducted whilst external rotation is applied. A clunk or grinding sound may indicate a labral tear.

Reference

Walsh DA. Shoulder evaluation in the throwing athlete. Sports Med. Update. 1989; 4: 24-27
Kibler WB. Specificity and sensitivity of the anterior slide test in throwing atheletes with superior glenoid labral tears. Arthroscopy. 1995; 11: 296-300.

Other Labral tests include:
- Compression rotation test
- Kocher's manoeuvre
- Anterior glide test

The Shoulder - Special Tests

SLAP LESIONS

The tests for long head of biceps pathology may be positive in the presence of SLAP lesions. Hence the Speed's and Yergason's test should be performed even though the specificity of each test on its own is considered low. The O'Brien's and Biceps load tests are considered more specific for SLAP lesions although the authors are not aware of any correlation between the presence of positive tests and the grading of a SLAP lesion.

O'Brien's Test:

Examiner stands behind the patient. Ask the patient to forward flex the affected arm to 90° with the elbow in full extension. The patient then adducts the arm 10° to 15° medial to the sagittal plane of the body. The arm is internally rotated so that the thumb points downward. Uniform downward force to the arm is applied by the examiner. With the arm in the same position, the palm is then fully supinated and uniform downward force applied. The test is considered positive if the patient's typical pain is elicited with forearm pronated and is reduced or eliminated with the forearm supinated. Pain or painful clicking within the glenohumeral joint is considered indicative of labral abnormality. Pain during this test localized to the acromioclavicular joint or on top of the shoulder may indicate acromioclavicular joint abnormality.

Reference:
O'Brien SJ, Pagnani MJ, Fealy S, et al: The active compression test: A new and effective test for diagnosing labral tears and acromioclavicular joint abnormality. Am J Sports Med 26:610 -613,1998

Biceps Load Test II:

With the patient supine, the examiner seated beside the patient, forearm in supination, elbow flexed to 90 degrees, the shoulder is elevated to 120 degrees in full external rotation. The patient is asked to flex the elbow against resistance. The test is positive if the patient feels pain on resisted elbow flexion or if the pain increases on resisted elbow flexion.

Reference
Kim SH, Ha KI, Ahn JH, et al: Biceps load test II: A clinical test for SLAP Lesions of the shoulder. Arthroscopy 17:160 -164, 2001

THORACIC OUTLET SYNDROME

Thoracic outlet syndrome is rarely a cause for isolated pains around the shoulder. However it should always be considered in patients with atypical pain distribution especially if it radiates distally into the forearm and is associated with vague neurological symptoms. The three commonly used tests are **Adson's, Wright's and Roos.** It should be remembered that these tests are often positive in asymptomatic normal patients.

ADSON'S TEST

With the patient sitting locate the radial pulse. Externally rotate, extend and slightly abduct the arm. Ask the patient to look towards the side of examination and take a deep breath. Abolition or a reduction in the pulse is a positive result.

Reference;

Adson AW and Coffey JR: Cervical rib: A method of anterior approach for relief of symptoms by division of the scalenus anticus. Ann Surg. 85:839-857, 1927.

The Shoulder - Special Tests

WRIGHT'S TEST

Abduct the arm to 90 degrees with external rotation whilst palpating the pulse. Again the abolition of the pulse is a positive test. This test is also called the Hyperabduction Test and provides a high false positive results.

Reference;
Wright IS. The neurovascular syndrome produced by hyperabduction of the arms. Am. Heart J. 29:1-19,1945.

ROOS TEST

The shoulder is abducted and the elbow flexed to 90 degrees. In this position the patient is asked to open and close the hands for three minutes. An inability to complete this exercise or reproduction of their symptoms indicates a positive result.

Reference;
Roos DB. Congenital anomalies associated with thoracic outlet syndrome. J. Surg. 132:771-778, 1976.

Technique
With the patient supine, one hand is placed on the posterior aspect of the shoulder whilst the other holds the humerus above the elbow.

The arm is fully abducted whilst external rotation is applied.

With the **anterior glide test** an anterosuperior force is applied at the elbow with the patient sitting.

The **compression rotation test** - the humeral head is pushed in the glenoid during internal and external rotation.

Clinical relevance
A clunk or grind is indicative of a tear in the labrum.

Reference
Walsh DA. Shoulder evaluation in the throwing athelete.
Sports Med. Update. 1989; 4: 24-27

Kibler WB. Specificity and sensitivity of the anterior slide test in throwing atheletes with superior glenoid labral tears.
Arthroscopy. 1995; 11: 296-300.

Other tests or signs:

Ludington's test	(long head of biceps)
Gilchrest sign	(bicipital tendinitis)
Lippman's test	(bicipital tendinitis)
Heuter's sign	(ruptured biceps)
"Empty can" test	(supraspinatus)
Codman's drop-arm test	(rotator cuff tear)
Wrights manoeuvre	(costoclavicular compression)
Allen test	(thoracic outlet syndrome)
Adson manoeuvre	(thoracic outlet syndrome)

The Shoulder - Clinical Cases

As with all other sections, to blindly perform all tests demonstrates a lack of understanding and clinical acumen. Adapt your examination as you proceed, based upon the patient's age and clinical findings as you examine them, a common example is described below.

Impingement in Young Adults

HISTORY

A 22-year-old man presents with a history of recurrent dislocation of his right (dominant) shoulder. This started following an incident whilst playing rugby 3 years previously in which he sustained a dislocation following a rough tackle. This was reduced in the accident unit within 6 hours using sedation. Following this he was supported in a board arm sling for 3 weeks and then commenced self-mobilisation. He was not referred for formal physiotherapy and was discharged from orthopaedic care at this stage.

He presented with further episodes of dislocation with decreasing force, all treated conservatively. He has had a course of physiotherapy specifically to strengthen the rotator cuff torn 2 years previously.

He is now 6 months following his fifth dislocation on the right side that was treated as previously. He cannot voluntarily dislocate his shoulder and between episodes of dislocation has no pain. He gets the feeling of instability when lifting objects above his head whilst at work as a warehouse man which has resulted in him giving up playing rugby for his local team.

EXAMINATION

On inspection he is a well-built man who tends to favour his left arm while undressing. He has no scars and no visible wasting. His neck and shoulder contours are normal.

Palpation relieves no specific areas of deformity or tenderness.

Forward flexion is limited actively to 100° completing an arc of 120° passively.

Extension again is limited to 40° both actively and passively in comparison to the other side.

Abduction is 100° actively with a normal rhythm and can be completed passively to 140°.

He has pain only at the extremes of movement.

He can hold the arm out vertically with normal deltoid contraction.

Adduction was again limited to 40°.

External rotation was limited to 40° by pain in both adduction and abduction of 90°.

The 'Apley Scratch Test' reiterated the degree of movement limitations previously found.

The power in all muscle groups was normal. As was sensation and peripheral circulation.

Impingement tests relieved a mildly positive impingement test. Speeds and Yergason's test were normal.

Anterior draw was positive grade 2 and apprehension was positive (worse at 90°).

The load and shift test was positive. The sulcus was negative, as were tests for posterior instability.

The Jobe relocation was strongly positive.

The Shoulder - Clinical Cases

RADIOLOGICAL ASSESSMENT

What plain films should be requested in the OPD?

Are there other radiological investigations that can help?

What are the benefits of Ultrasound Scanning?

MRI can be ordered with or without contrast.

FRCS TYPE QUESTIONS:

1. Why is the impingement test positive with instability?

2. Do immobilisation, formal physiotherapy and arthroscopic washout affect the outcome in the first dislocation and subsequent dislocations?

3. What further investigations would you perform? Why? What do you expect to see?

4. What procedures if any would you consider in this patient? What are the advantages and disadvantages of each procedure? What would you warn the patient pre-operatively?

The Shoulder - Clinical Cases

Shoulder cases

Young

Instability

Middle age

Frozen shoulder
Calcific tendinitis
Impingement

Older

Rotator cuff tear
Arthritis

INSTABILITY TESTS

Patient sitting initially arm on the lap
Any voluntary component? 'Can you put your shoulder out'
Anterior   - anterior draw
               - load and shift test
               - measure degree of translation
               - apprehension test ($90°$ abduction and external rotation)
Inferior   - sulcus sign

Lie patient down
Posterior   - load and shift
               - push pull test (Norwood)
Relocation test (Jobe) and release
Labral tests and Kocher manoeuvre

Examination of the Brachial Plexus
Mr Alex A J Kocheta FRCS
Specialist Registrar, Orthopaedics
Mr David Ford MB BS, FRCS, FRCS Ed (Orth)
Consultant Orthopaedic Hand Surgeon.
Mr Simon Pickard FRCS (Tr and Orth)
Consultant Orthopaedic Hand Surgeon

Principles of the Examination

Usually, the brachial plexus is damaged following open or closed trauma in the adult or obstetric trauma in the infant. The latter is outside the scope of this work.

Plexus injuries frequently involve only parts of the plexus and may be at any level (or several levels) within it. The most proximal injuries are preganglionic root avulsions and are associated with, upper motor nerve signs in the legs and pseudomeningocoele and late development of syrinx of the cord. If involving the T1 root then a Horner's syndrome may be present.

The goal of examination is to discern a pattern of injury that relates to an anatomical level within the brachial plexus, whether it be the roots, the trunks, the cords or the terminal branches alone. From this information and the degree of dysfunction, a treatment plan can be formulated.

To facilitate this, it is necessary to be familiar with the anatomy of the plexus and to have in mind an examination routine that is both logical and methodical. This allows an anatomical picture of the injury to be built up. The technique described below is a **proximal to distal routine** that examines the roots in order from C5 to T1 and also each of the major branches.

IMPORTANT POINTS OF CLINICAL ANATOMY
The roots of the plexus lie between the scalenus anterior and medius muscles.
The trunks lie in the posterior triangle of the neck.
The divisions of the trunks lie behind the clavicle and at the outer border of the first rib. The divisions form the cords, the cords lie in the upper axilla.
This anatomical arrangement should be borne in mind when assessing injuries around the neck and shoulder.

The numbers 3 and 5 should be remembered when considering the branches.
There are 3 branches from the 5 roots.
The 3 cords give rise to the following numbers of branches:
> 3 from the lateral cord,
> 5 from the posterior cord and
> 5 from the medial cord.
The exception is the single branch from the upper trunk.

The root values decrease as one passes down the plexus from the lateral cord (C5,6,7) to the posterior cord (C5,6,7,8) to the medial cord (C8,T1).

Again the exception to this is the 90% of individuals who receive C6 & 7 fibres into the ulnar nerve (medial cord) via a branch from the lateral cord. These fibres supply flexor carpi ulnaris in the forearm.

The stellate ganglion also has a root value of T1 and may be denervated in lower plexus root avulsions. It is from here that the sympathetic supply to the eye arises and if interrupted gives rise to a Horner's syndrome (ptosis, miosis, apparent enophthalmos and absence of sweating over the ipsilateral face).

The vertebral arteries lie anteriorly to the roots and supply radicular arteries, particularly around the C5, 6 and 7 roots. Avulsion at this level may be associated with a Brown-Séquard syndrome in up to 5% of cases. This cord hemisection syndrome involves:-
> ipsilateral total sensory loss at the level of the lesion,
> ipsilateral dorsal column loss distally (loss of proprioception and vibration sense) as well as
> ipsilateral motor weakness.
On the contralateral side there is spinothalamic impairment (loss of pain and temperature sensibility) distal to the lesion.

Other vascular injuries are not uncommon:-
> 15% of supraclavicular distraction lesions are associated with subclavian artery rupture.
> 30% of infraclavicular injuries are associated with axillary artery rupture.

Examination of the Brachial Plexus

The trapezius muscle is not innervated by the brachial plexus but by the spinal accessory nerve (C3,4). The trapezius is, however, assessed as it often gives some shoulder function and it or its nerve may be transferred e.g. to deltoid.

Old obstetric brachial palsies may show signs of cord damage such as a small ipsilateral foot and gait problems.

It is important to distinguish preganglionic (i.e. intradural avulsions of the ventral and dorsal spinal nerve roots proximal to the dorsal root ganglion) injuries from postganglionic. The latter are ruptures of the proper spinal nerve distal to the dorsal root ganglion. The importance of differentiation is in treatment and later recovery.

Preganglionic avulsions tend to recover poorly and are not amenable to reconstruction whereas the converse may be true of postganglionic lesions.

Preganglionic avulsions will require nerve transfers (neurotization) or muscle transfers. Cord injury is obviously more likely with preganglionic injury.

A striking feature of preganglionic avulsion is the history of immediate pain from the time of injury.

MOTOR TESTING

When assessing motor power, the MRC grading system is used. For a grade to be given, the joint being examined must have a full range of passive movement.

Where active movement of the joint is possible, the muscle must be able to pull the joint through a full range otherwise a lower grade should be allocated, e.g. when examining the elbow for flexion power, the biceps must be able to flex the elbow completely from the extended position against gravity to score a 3. If it cannot do this, despite being able to flex the elbow a little against gravity then a score of 2 or 1 should be given.

MRC GRADES 0-5:

Grade 0:	No discernible flicker of contraction.
Grade 1:	Flicker of contraction only.
Grade 2:	The muscle contracts sufficiently to move the joint through its full range of motion in a plane perpendicular to gravity.
Grade 3:	The muscle contracts to move the joint through its full range of motion against the action of gravity.
Grade 4:	The muscle contracts to move the joint through its full range of motion against some external resistance.
Grade 5:	The muscle contracts to move the joint through its full range of motion with normal power.

Grade 4 may be subdivided into:-

4-	(slight resistance),
4	(moderate resistance) and
4+	(strong resistance)

Anatomy of the Brachial Plexus

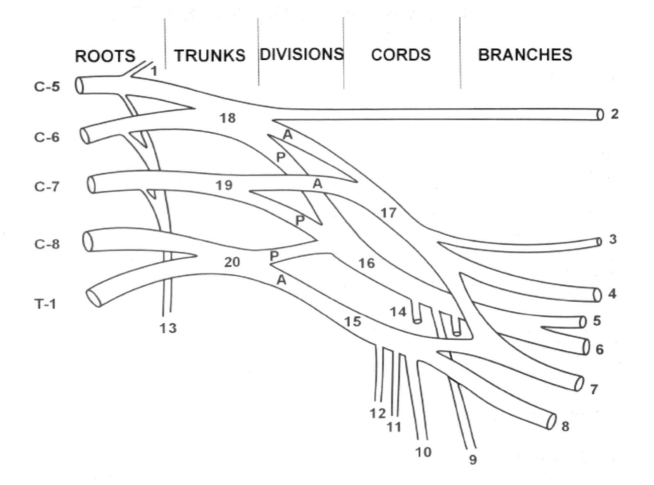

BRACHIAL PLEXUS

1	Dorsal scapular		11	Medial brachial nerve
2	Suprascapular		12	Medial pectoral nerve
3	Lateral pectoral nerve		13	Long thoracic
4	Musculocutaneous nerve		14	Upper & lower subscapular
5	Axillary nerve		15	Medial cord
6	Radial nerve		16	Posterior cord
7	Median nerve		17	Lateral cord
8	Ulnar nerve		18	Upper trunk
9	Thoracodorsal nerve		19	Middle trunk
10	Medial antebrachial nerve		20	Lower trunk

Examination of the Brachial Plexus

Systematic Examination of the Brachial Plexus

The routine of look, feel, move can still be applied to this situation.

Feeling should incorporate palpation for muscle wasting and sensory testing.
Moving incorporates an assessment of tone and power testing (MRC grade).
The reflexes should also be checked.

Special tests for peripheral nerve function may be appropriate.

INSPECTION

The patient is stripped to the waist to allow visualisation of both upper limbs and the torso musculature.

Careful inspection is performed for old wounds, both traumatic and surgical. The axilla is not neglected. The muscle masses of the back (latissimus dorsi and trapezius), the scapular region (rhomboids medially, supra and infraspinatus over the scapular blade and teres major and minor laterally) are noted. Anteriorly the pectoralis major mass is assessed for wasting.

The upper limb is inspected from the shoulder to the finger tips beginning with the deltoid, passing down the arm (biceps, brachialis and triceps) to the forearm (mobile wad and extensor compartment as well as the flexor compartment).

The hand is checked for intrinsic muscle wasting between the metacarpals as well as the thenar and hypothenar eminences. Trophic changes and ulcers may be observed in the digits.

Any evidence of other injuries in the upper limbs is also noted as there may frequently be associated long bone fractures due to the high kinetic energy transfer that often takes place at the time of injury.

Surgical treatments may have been carried out if the plexus lesion is chronic and muscle transfer scars, joint fusions and amputations should be noted as well as any prostheses.

A malunited clavicular fracture may be noted.

The resting position of the limb should be noted. Any fixed deformity is commented upon e.g. clawing of the hand, fixed internal rotation of the shoulder, extension of the elbow etc.

Examination of the Brachial Plexus

PALPATION

The chest, back and upper limb musculature are felt to assess remaining bulk.

Sensation is assessed by first asking the patient to outline the area of abnormality. Objective assessment is then carried out from the insensate area to the sensate. The direction may be reversed if the area is hypersensitive. Light touch is tested with gentle digital pressure and pin-prick with a neurological pin.

The dermatomal innervation may be a little variable but it is generally held that:-
>C5 innervates the lateral arm,
>C6 the lateral forearm and thumb,
>C7 the middle finger,
>C8 the little finger and ulnar border of the hand and
>T1 the medial forearm.

Sensation above the clavicles and acromion is generally C4 with C3 but this area is more variable.

The limb should also be examined for specific peripheral sensory nerve lesions highlighting cord lesions.

Axilliary nerve.	innervates a small patch of skin over the distal deltoid belly and insertion.
Radial nerve	innervates the skin of the lateral arm below the Axillary nerve territory and along a thin strip of posteroradial forearm to the dorsum of the first web space.
Medial cutaneous nerve	of the arm innervates the skin above the elbow medially.
Musculocutaneous nerve.	The continuation of this as the lateral cutaneous nerve of the forearm innervates the lateral forearm to the wrist.
Ulnar nerve.	Innervates the ulnar one-and-a-half digits and the ulnar third of the hand both dorsally and volarly.
Median nerve.	Innervates the radial three-and-a-half digits of the hand on the volar aspect and the dorsum of the same distal phalanges.

Examination of the Brachial Plexus

MOVEMENT

Asking the patient to relax the limb, grasping the hand as though to shake it and passively moving the wrist, elbow and shoulder, allows assessment of tone. Increased tone indicates an upper motor neurone lesion and decreased a lower.

It is important to assess the passive range of movement of all the upper limb joints in every plane prior to assessing power. If this is not done it is not possible to accurately grade the power of the muscle groups according to the MRC system.

One should now individually assess the power of each muscle in the upper limbs as far as is practicable.

A system based on knowledge of the anatomy of the brachial plexus is necessary to avoid missing any lesions and fully assess the extent of involvement at each level of the plexus.

Each test is designed to isolate the intended muscle and as far as is possible to only test its action across a single joint.

The order of examination is generally myotomal but slight variations from the strict order are included to improve the fluidity of the examination and to prevent excessive movements of the examiner from the front to the back of the patient.

The first eight muscles are tested with examiner behind the patient. Each muscle is tested for a visual and palpable contraction as well as an MRC power grading (0-5). Suggested commands to the patients after the upper limbs have been placed in the appropriate position are given in inverted commas.

Examination of the Brachial Plexus

Trapezius. (Spinal accessory C3,4)

The patient is asked to shrug the shoulders. The contraction of trapezius superiorly can be seen and felt.

"Shrug your shoulders."

To assess the lower fibres, the patient is asked to stand in front of a wall, flex the shoulders to 90°, extend the elbows and pronate the forearms whilst pushing hard on the wall. The lower fibres of trapezius are seen and felt to contract.

A type of scapular winging (mainly inferior) may ensue from lower trapezius palsy.

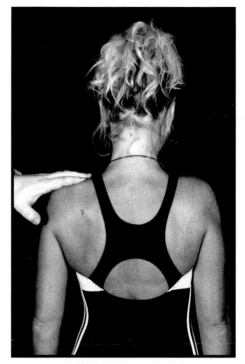

Serratus anterior. (Long thoracic n. C5,6,7)

From the same position the patient is asked to continue pushing into the wall.

"Push into the wall as hard as you can."

True medial scapular winging is indicative of serratus anterior palsy.

Changes of position e.g. with the shoulders flexed 45° and the forearms supinated or the shoulders flexed to 120° and the forearms crossed in front of the face may bring out subtle winging more clearly than the standard position.

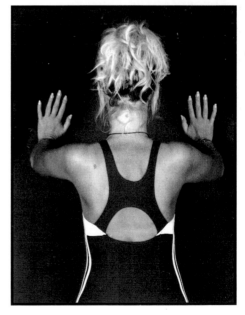

Fig.54 Testing Serratus Anterior (Long Thoracic nerve; C5, C6, C7). Now ask them to push against a wall, note any winging of the scapula.

Examination of the Brachial Plexus

Rhomboids. (Dorsal scapular n. C5)

The patient is asked to brace the shoulders back. The contraction of the rhomboids medial to the scapula can be seen and felt.

"Push against my hand"

It is easy to confuse trapezius contraction with rhomboid.

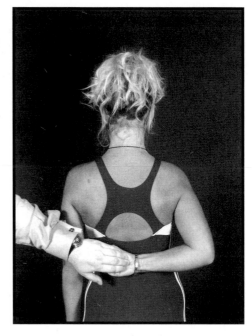

Fig.55 Testing the Rhomboids (Dorsal Scapular nerve C5).

Supraspinatus (Suprascapular n. C5,6)

With the examiner again behind, the patient's shoulder is placed in internal rotation with the thumb pointing medially and is abducted 20° in the line of the scapula. Further abduction in the same plane is resisted.

"Keep your arm where it's been put."

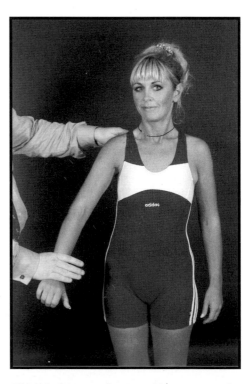

*Fig.56 Supraspinatus (Suprascapular nerve; **C5**, C6). Ask the patient to abduct the slightly forward flexed arm with the hand pronated against resistance.*

Examination of the Brachial Plexus

Infraspinatus. (Suprascapular n. C5,6)
The shoulder is placed in adduction and neutral rotation with the elbow flexed 90°. External rotation is resisted at the forearm whilst the elbow is prevented from abducting with the other hand.

"Push your hands outwards, away from each other."

Deltoid (Axillary Nerve C5,6)
The shoulder is abducted to 90° with the elbow flexed. The anterior and middle fibres can be seen. Both sides are usually tested simultaneously.

"Keep your arms where they have been put."

Resisted retraction of the arm from this position highlights the posterior fibres.

"Now push your elbows backwards."

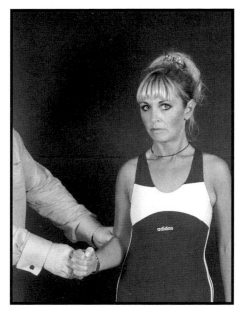

*Fig.57 Infraspinatus (Suprasacpular nerve; **C5**, C6). Elbow by your side push your wrist out against my hand.*

Latissimus dorsi (Thoracodorsal n. (C6,7,8)
With the arm abducted to 90°, resisted adduction will highlight the muscle belly half way down the thoracic cage laterally.

"Pull your elbow down to your side."

The muscle also contracts on coughing.

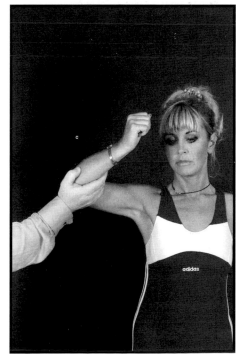

*Fig.58 Testing Latissimus Dorsi (Thoracodorsal nerve; C6, **C7**, C8)*

Teres major (Suprascapular n. C5,6,7)
This smaller muscle belly is also highlighted by the above test. It lies above the latissimus dorsi.

Examination of the Brachial Plexus

THE FOLLOWING EXAMINATIONS ARE MADE WITH THE EXAMINER IN FRONT OF THE PATIENT:

Pectoralis major.

The clavicular head (Lateral pectoral n. **C5**,6) may be examined with the examiner in front of the patient. The shoulder is abducted to 100° and externally rotated 80°. The patient is asked to push the arm forward.

"Push against me."

The sternal head (Lateral and medial pectoral n.'s C6,**7**,8) is examined by resisted shoulder adduction from 30° of abduction.

Biceps Brachii (Musculocutaneous Nerve C5,6)

With the shoulder adducted, the forearm should be supinated and the elbow flexed against resistance.

"Pull my hand towards you."

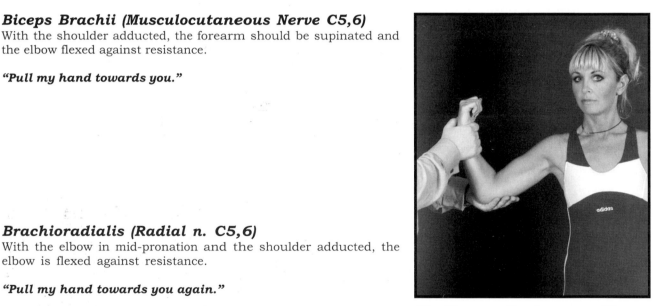

Brachioradialis (Radial n. C5,6)

With the elbow in mid-pronation and the shoulder adducted, the elbow is flexed against resistance.

"Pull my hand towards you again."

Fig.59   Testing   Biceps (Musculocutaneous nerve; C5, C6).

Triceps (Radial n. C6,7,8)

The patient's forearm should now be pronated, the shoulder flexed 45° and the elbow extended.

"Now push me away."

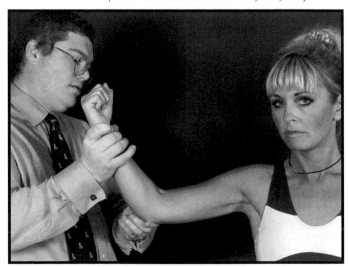

*Fig.60 Testing Triceps (Radial nerve C6, **C7**, C8).*

Examination of the Brachial Plexus

Supinator (Radial n. C6)
With the elbow extended and the forearm pronated, the patient's hand is grasped as though for a hand shake and he is asked to supinate against resistance.

"Try to turn your hand over."

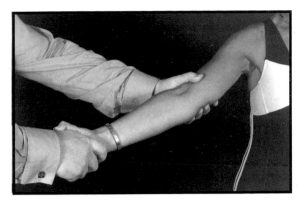

Fig.61 Testing Supinator (Radial nerve; C6,C7).

Extensor Carpi Radialis Longus Brevis (Radial n. C5,6)
The patient's elbow is flexed 90° with the shoulder abducted and the forearm pronated 45°. The wrist is extended. The examiner's hand exerts pressure over the dorsum of the index MCPJ.

"Keep your hand where it is."

Extensor Carpi Ulnaris (Posterior interosseous n. C7,8)
From the same initial position as previously, pressure is exerted over the little MCPJ.

"Keep your hand where it is."

Extensor Digitorum (Posterior interosseous n. C7,8)
The palm of the patient's hand is supported and pressure is applied across the dorsum of the extended proximal phalanges of the fingers.

"Keep your fingers out straight."

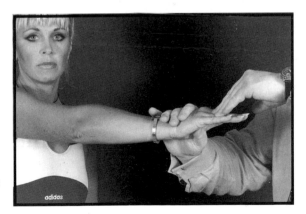

Fig.62 Testing Extensor Digitorum (Posterior Interosseous nerve; **C7**, C8)

Extensor Pollicis Brevis (Posterior interosseous n. C7,8)
Resisted extension of the thumb MCPJ. The tendon is palpable just to the ulnar side of abductor pollicis longus at the snuffbox.

Extensor Pollicis Longus (Posterior interosseous n. C7,8)
Resisted extension of the thumb interphalangeal joint. The tendon is palpable on the ulnar side of the snuffbox.

Examination of the Brachial Plexus

Abductor Pollicis Longus (Posterior interosseous n. C7,8)

The thumb is abducted against resistance. The APL tendon is palpated on the radial side of the anatomical snuffbox.

"Push your thumb up against mine."

Pronator Teres (Median n. C6,7)

With the elbow flexed, resisted pronation highlights this muscle which can be palpated medial to the cubital fossa.

"Turn your hand against mine."

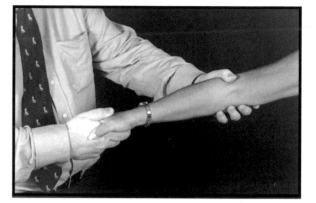

Fig.63 Testing Pronator Terres (Median nerve; **C6***, C7).*

Flexor Carpi Radialis (Median n. C6,7)

Ask the patient to make a fist and then to flex the wrist. Resist with radial-sided pressure.

Flexor Digitorum Superficialis (Median n. C7,8,1)

Ask the patient to perform resisted flexion of the individual PIPJ's.

Flexor Digitorum Profundus to Index & Middle Fingers (Anterior interosseous n. C7,8)

Fix the middle phalanx in extension and ask the patient to perform resisted flexion of the DIPJ.

Flexor Pollicis Longus (Anterior interosseous n. C7,8)

Fix the proximal phalanx of the thumb in extension and ask the patient to perform resisted flexion of the IPJ.

Abductor Pollicis Brevis (Median n. T1)

Place the patient's hand into supination and ask him to abduct the thumb against resistance. Many patients have trouble understanding the exact position required and therefore I tend to place my finger above the thumb and ask them to

"touch my finger with your thumb".

Examination of the Brachial Plexus

Flexor Carpi Ulnaris (Ulnar n. C7,8,T1)
This is best tested indirectly by asking the patient to abduct the little finger against resistance.

Abductor digiti minimi arises from the pisiform bone in part and the FCU tendon contracts to stabilise the pisiform even if the ADM is paralysed. It can be seen and felt to contract on the ulnar side of the volar aspect of the wrist.

This obviously also tests the ADM (Ulnar n. **T1**)

Flexor Digitorum Profundus to the Ring and Little Fingers (Ulnar n. C7,8)
Fix the middle phalanx in extension and ask the patient to perform resisted flexion of the DIPJ.

The Second Palmar Interosseous (Ulnar n. T1)
This can easily be tested by using the "card test". The patient is asked to flex the little and ring fingers into the palm whilst extending the index and middle fingers. A sheet of thin card is then held between the index and middle fingers by adduction of the index. The examiner opposes this exactly and a test by confrontation is carried out by the patient attempting to pull the card from the examiner's grip.

Froment's test
This is carried out to test the Adductor Pollicis (Ulnar n. C8,T1).
The patient is asked to grasp a piece of card in the first web space, between the extended thumb and the radial border of the hand. If the IPJ flexes then the test is positive as the patient is attempting to hold the card using the flexor pollicis longus rather than the paralysed adductor pollicis.

The entire upper limb and brachial plexus have now been examined for sensation and power.

Further investigation usually comprises MR scanning and possibly exploration.
Myelography was used extensively in the past but less so now.
Electrophysiological testing is used both preoperatively and intraoperatively.

The Spine

Mr Jay Trivedi MCh Orth, FRCS (Orth)
Consultant Spinal Surgeon

Examination of the spine is best subdivided into anatomical regions - cervical, thoracic and lumbar. Examination of the spine is a test of one's knowledge of anatomy. One must have a thorough awareness of the dermatomal and myotomal innervation of the upper and lower limbs. Without this knowledge it is fruitless to proceed as almost invariably, you will be asked to perform a neurological assessment on the patient.

THE CERVICAL SPINE.

Common Clinical Cases

1. Cervical disc herniation with a radiculopathy
2. Cervical stenosis with myeolpathy. Know the difference between a radiculopathy and a myelopathy. Radiculopathy implies a lower motor neurone pathology (absent reflex at that level with associated sensory and motor impairment), whereas myelopathy is an upper motor neurone lesion (brisk reflexes below the level of involvement)
3. Rarely traumatic conditions (torticollis from Atlantoaxial subluxation or congential torticollis)

The first and often most helpful clues occur when you see the patient.

Age - young age more commonly associated with acute disc herniations, trauma and congenital disorders, and an older patient with a degenerative or (rarely in the exam setting) a neoplastic process (myelopathy). However, inflammatory conditions, such as rheumatoid arthritis or ankylosing spondylitis can occur at any age.

Are they standing, sitting or lying down?

Do their clothes give anything away? Velcro fastening on a blouse may imply loss of dexterity and difficulty in doing fine tasks.

Are there any orthotics on view? We have mentioned this before but do you really know the difference between the varieties of walking aids and what they may mean, such as a standing frame and pulpit rollator?

Introduce yourself - It is your first point of contact.

General Examination

Begin with a quick assessment of higher cranial function especially in the elderly. Beware of the patient who may have had a stroke in the past with resultant hemiparesis. This may influence your neurological examination. Check for any speech disorders. These should be obvious by talking to the patient.

Assess the facial nerve by examining for facial weakness or asymmetry. Ask the patient to blow his cheeks (buccinator) and clench his teeth (masseter).

Ask the patient to stand. Is he or she unsteady on his feet? (posterior column dysfunction, peripheral neuropathy).
Next, examine the patient's gait. Is it a broad based ataxic gait? Is it spastic? (Does he or she have difficulty in clearance during swing). The latter may suggest cord compression and myelopathy.

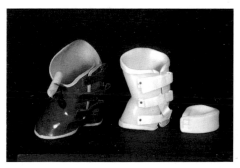

Fig.65 Neck collars, leather block and spinal corsets give you clues regarding diagnosis and likely physical signs to help focus your examination.

The Spine

Ask the patient to take their top off. It is quite acceptable to maintain a lady's modesty by keeping the bra in place. Does the patient fumble with the buttons suggesting some loss of dexterity? (myelopathy).

Look

Look for any cervical orthoses. Common ones include a soft collar, a Philadelphia collar and a halo-vest (Fig 65). If they have a collar on, ask if this may be removed but it is unlikely you will be given an Allen key and spanner to remove a Halo frame. If they do have a frame on, then describe this, with regards to the number and position of the pins and their condition i.e clean, crusted or infected.

From the front:

Does the patient have a torticollis? This is characterized by the "cock robin" posture with the head tilted to one side. Observe whether the sternomastoid muscle is prominent on the side of the tilt (as in congenital torticollis) or on the opposite side (as in atlanto-axial subluxation). Is there a hypolasia of one half of the face suggestive of long standing torticollis?

Can you see the incision from an anterior approach to spine? Does the patient have or is there a scar from a tracheostomy? Are there any lumps in the supraclavicular fossa? Is there a goitre? Is there Horner's Syndrome? Look for any asymmetry in the level of the shoulders (Sprengel's Shoulder, Scoliosis).

From the side:

Observe the normal cervical lordosis or the lack of it. Is there an exaggerated thoracic kyphosis?

From behind:

In a long haired patient, lift the hair out of the way. Are there any scars or bumps that need closer inspection and later palpation?

Feel

Most palpation in the cervical examination can be done from behind and is often less tiring for the patient, and easier for you, if they are sitting down. Use a pattern of starting at the occiput and work your way down over the erector spinae and spinous processes.
Remember the most prominent spinous process belongs to T1. Feel for tenderness and alignment of the spinous processes. Descend into the thoracic spine at least as far caudally as the mid-thoracic area.
Then work your way out, bilaterally, coming around and over the trapezius into the supraclavicular fossae.

Be gentle, do not throttle the patient!

Feel the top of the manubrium sterni and advance cranially towards the thyroid gland; feel the lobes. and continue upwards.

Remember the hyoid bone is a landmark for C3-4 level.

Assess the tension in the sternomastoid muscle.

The Spine

Move

Always start with active movement to avoid any unpleasant yelps from a patient. You can ask the patient to put a tongue depressor in their mouth to act as a guide to the range but this is not strictly necessary.

Ask the patient to hold their head in a comfortable position; does this differ from neutral?
Then **"chin on chest"** for forward flexion, usually about 75 degrees but this normally varies with age. (Fig 66)

Then **"look up at the ceiling"** for extension, usually about 50 degrees so the whole range of motion is about 125 degrees. (Fig 66)

Then lateral flexion, **"put your right ear on your right shoulder"** and the opposite for the left. Look at the rise of the shoulder and compare sides, the range of motion is usually about 90 degrees (Fig 67)
"Put your right chin on your right shoulder" will test rotation which is just short of 90 degrees so compare the shoulder shrug that should occur on both sides.(Fig 68)

Do not forget **Spurling's Test** for radiculopathy. The patient's head is flexed laterally and extended. This narrows the nerve root foramina on the concave side and reproduces their radicular pain.

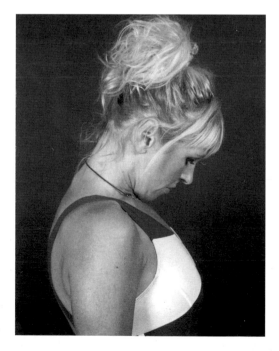 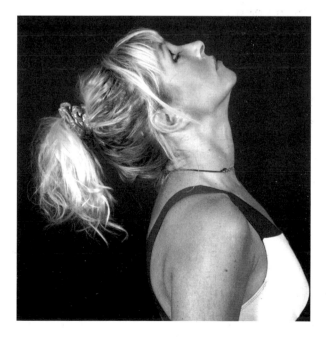

Fig. 66 .Flexion and extension of the cervical spine mainly occurs between C3 to C7 with most movement at the C2-3, C3-4 and C4-5 vertebral spaces.

The Spine

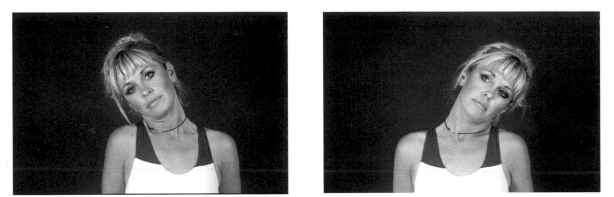

Fig.67. Lateral flexion of the cervical spine.

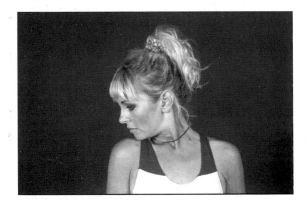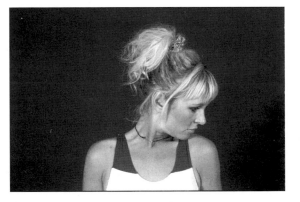

Fig.68. Rotation of the cervical spine most movement occurring at the atlantoaxial joints (C1-2).

Neurology

It is not acceptable to just test the upper limb neurology, find no lesion and stop there. A complete neurological examination of upper and lower limbs is required but we will cover the lower limbs in the lumbar spine section.

Remember - ***tone, power, sensation, coordination, proprioception and reflexes.***

Are the upper limbs held flaccid or is there a spastic posture?

Power can be assessed rapidly by..., **shrug your shoulders** (spinal accessory nerve), **lift your arms from your side** (C5), **bend your elbows and push against me** (C7), **now pull towards you** (C5/6), **cock your wrist stiff and do not let me bend it** (C6/7), **grip my finger tightly** (C7/8), **open your hand, spread your fingers in a fan, do not let me close them** (C8/T1)...."

Practice the patter and get a rhythm - each test is examining a level and power can be marked on theMRC scale.

Sensation, classically, can be soft touch, deep pressure or pin prick. To repeat all three may be seen as time wasting and demonstrate a poor grasp of the purpose of examination. Although soft touch is easy to perform, insist where possible to test with a pin prick. Have a very clear dermatome map in mind i.e., C5 (regimental badge area of the shoulder), C6 (lateral aspect of the forearm), C7 (anterior distal middle finger), C8 anterior distal aspect little finger and T1 (medial side of elbow). Remember the autonomous zone of a nerve which is an area of skin supplied solely by that nerve.

The Spine

Coordination and proprioception expose a central pathology, chronic alcohol abuse, cord compression etc.

Adapt your examination to fit the patient, concentrate on aspects that are going to help you make a reasoned diagnosis.

Reflexes - again marry in your mind that each reflex is testing root values.

Reflex	Root value	Technique
The biceps reflex	C5	Flex the elbow, and with a finger on the biceps tendon in the cubital fossa tap lightly with your hammer. (Fig 69)
The brachioradialis reflex	C6	Tap the tendon over the radial border of the distal forearm with the elbow flexed and neutrally rotated. (Fig 70)
The triceps jerk	C7	Tap the triceps tendon proximal to the elbow with the elbow flexed. (Fig 71)

Reflexes can be difficult to demonstrate and subtle differences can be overlooked. Remember they can be enhanced by "re-enforcement." Ask the patient to clench his teeth or clasp his hands tightly together and then attempt to elicit the reflex.
Also, in the hyper reflexive patient, put the hammer down and tap using just your finger.

Fig. 69. The Biceps reflex (C5).

Fig. 70. The Brachioradialis reflex (C6).

Fig. 71 The Triceps Reflex (C7).

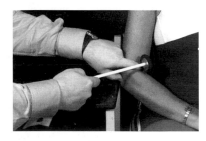
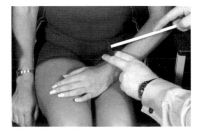
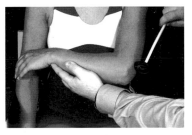

The Spine

SPECIAL CASES.

The **cervical rib** may be presented to you as a hand case or a neck examination, so be warned. The more poignant case will have vascular changes unilaterally in the hand with cold, white, mottled or bluish discoloration of the fingers, along with trophic changes in the nails and in advanced cases trophic ulceration.. Do not be caught out by **Raynaud's** which is more often bilateral. Remember Raynaud has a disease, symptoms, signs and phenomena named after him.

Feel the radial pulse, apply gentle traction to the arm and see if the pulse character, volume or signal is altered. Compare sides. Hold the arm across the body, feel the radial pulse and ask the patient to look towards you and take a deep breath, again assess both sides and compare any alteration.

Finally listen for a bruit with a stethoscope in the supraclavicular fossa.

Cord compression and Myelopathy.

This is characterized by the presence of upper motor neurone signs below the level of compression (brisk tendon reflexes with or without clonus, absent superficial relexes and up going plantars). Remember that at the level of compression there will be lower motor neurone signs (absent tendon jerk and possible sensory impairment).

Tests for cervical myelopathy.

Hoffmann's sign - flick the terminal phalanx of the middle finger into extension suddenly and watch to see if the index finger and thumb flex involuntarily. The Hoffman's sign may be construed to be the equivalent of a Babinski response of the upper limbs. It is a very sensitive test for myelopathy.

Dynamic Hoffmann's test - the same flick as above, but get the patient to flex extend the neck at the same time.

Finger escape sign - The patient is asked to stretch his hands in front of him or her. The fingers of the hands should be closely adducted. When the test is positive the little finger drifts into abduction.

Finger fatigue test - The patient is asked to open and close his/her fists quickly. A patient with myelopathy soon fatigues doing this.

These tests demonstrate cortico-spinal tract dysfunction.

Lhermitte's sign is positive if flexion-extension of the neck produces an "electric shock" like sensation along the spine. (Fig 72)

Clonus occurs when the foot is rapidly brought up into dorsiflexion from a plantar position. It is counted as normal if there are two or three beats; more than this indicates an abnormality.

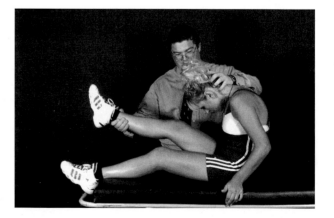

Fig. 72. Lhermitte's Test. Be gentle especially in the elderly, rheumatoid or ankylosing spondilitis patient!

Finally, in the cervical spine, complete your examination by a quick assessment of the carpal tunnel (Phalen's test and Tinel's sign) and the cubital tunnel. Also quickly put both shoulders through an active range of movement to pick up any concomitant shoulder pathology.

The Spine

THE THORACIC AND LUMBAR SPINE

Common Clinical Cases

1.   Lumbar disc herniation with radicular symptoms and signs
2.   Lumbar spinal canal stenosis
3.   Ankylosing spondylitis
4.   Thoracic cord compression (thoracic disc herniation, rarely tumors)
5.   Paediatric cases (Scoliosis and spondylolisthesis)

On seeing the patient for the first time many clues and possibilities should come to mind.
Age again is a vital clue e.g
Adolescent: Idiopathic scoliosis or spondylolisthesis
Adult: Think of lumbar disc herniation, ankylosing spondylitis
Elderly: Spinal stenosis.

Ask permission to undress the patient. In the exam atmosphere, most patients have been asked to dress appropriately to allow examination and more often than not are already prepared so time is not wasted. If they need to undress, assess how easy this is for them.

Ask them to stand. Does the patient stand with the hip and knee flexed on one side suggestive of sciatic irritation from a disc herniation? Is there a stoop? (spinal stenosis). Is there a marked thoracic kyphosis from ankylosing spondylitis?

Observe the gait.

Gait	Possible Diagnosis
Antalgic	Sciatica
High stepping gait	Foot drop from disc herniation, neuropathy, spinal stcnosis
Spastic	Myelopathy from cord compression
Ataxic or broad based	Myelopathy from cord compression
Normal but the spine stooped	Spinal stenosis

Ask the patient, as a quick screening test, to "tiptoe" walk, assessing S1 level and "heel" walk for L5 level assessment. If possible ask the patient to squat and then get up from a squatted position (L2, L3, L4) Then perform the Trendlenberg test to assess for hip abductor weakness.

Look;

This has two phases in the back exam - standing and sitting.

Standing, where leg length discrepancies and joint contractures may affect the posture of the spine.

Sitting, where any pelvic obliquity and spinal deformity is solely the result of a spinal etiology.

From the front - look for an obvious leaning posture. Look for any asymmetry in the shoulder height suggestive of a scoliosis. Can the patient maintain a horizontal gaze?

The Spine

From the side - is there a thoracotomy scar? Does this mean an anterior approach to the thoracic spine? Can you see a kyphosis? Does there appear to be a normal lumbar lordosis or has it flattened?

Remember, females and some racial groups can have an increase in lumbar lordosis. Exaggerated lumbar lordosis maybe associated with a hip pathology such as a long established bilateral DDH.

From the back (fig 73) - Once again assess for any asymmetry in the level of shoulders. Look for any abnormal skin pigmentation or cafe au lait spots suggestive of neurofibromatosis. Remember to count them - having up to 4 is counted as normal.

Is there a visual appearance of a scoliosis?

Is there a hair patch in the lumbar region, the so called Fawn's beard suggestive of spina bifida?

Has someone already been here and left a surgical scar?

Is the pelvis level or is there a pelvic obliquity? If there is one remember to look for any leg length discrepancy and also seat the patient on a couch to see if the pelvis levels out.

Are the waist creases balanced and equal? A flattened or obliterated waist crease on one side and an exaggerated crease on the other, is highly suggestive of a lumbar scoliosis.

Are the creases in the popliteal fossae at the the same level? A difference in the level may suggest a leg length discrepancy.

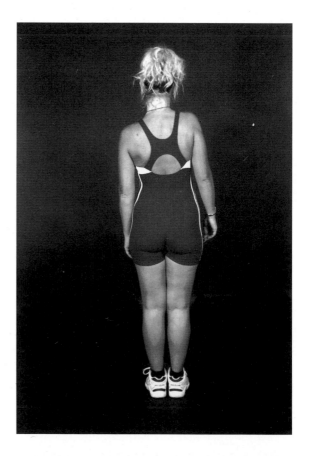

Fig. 73. Standing view from behind. Look for symmetry at different levels i.e. shoulders, pelvis, popliteal fossa and heel. Ask yourself is the head inline above the pelvis? If a scoliosis is present start describing it and look for costal impingement and a rib hump.

The Spine

Now concentrate on the spine itself.

Imagine a line running down from the occiput, the so called plumb line. Does it pass through the natal cleft? If not assess how far away from the midline does it pass. Does the spine deviate from this line?

Curves can always be described as convex left or concave right but, under pressure, an error can be made. Try just saying apex right or left to describe the curve. Ask the patient to gently bend forward the so called Adam's Position. In this position any scoliosis if present is more obvious as is a rib prominence if present. In the Adam's position ask the patient to rotate to the right and then left and remark on the change in the shape of the spine and rib prominence. A flexible curve may correct considerably on this side bend exercise.

In a younger child a similar assessment of the flexibility of the curve can be obtained by vertically suspending the child gently by holding it under its arms. Remember to take the mother into confidence prior to doing this or even get the mother to do this while you observe the child's back.

Ask the patient to sit on the edge of the bench, feet off the floor. With the pelvis level, does the curve correct?

Feel.

Feel the bony anatomy. Work down from the top. Feel for any tenderness and palpable gaps. The latter may suggest a high grade spondylolisthesis.

If comfortable then percuss the spine with the ulnar border of your fist.

Move.

Active first.

"Touch your toes" (fig 74) - often they cannot get down that far, so how far do the hands get down - mid thigh, knees or mid shin?

Remember this movement is a mass motion of not only lumbar and thoracic activity but also of hip flexion.

A more exact measure of spinal flexion is to use the **modified Schober's test.** The test uses two fixed points. With the patient standing, mark a point 10cm cephalad and 5cm caudal from the posterior-superior iliac spine (dimple of Venus). Now ask the patient to flex forwards and measure the excursion between the two points.

Normally this about 6-7cm.

Less than 5cm is suggestive of restricted flexion.
e.g. Ankylosing spondylitis

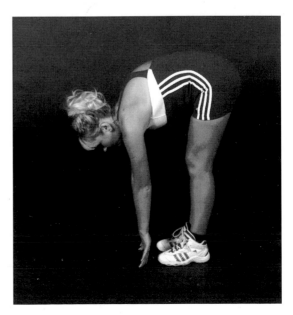

Fig. 74. Touch your toes. Not only look for the overall arc of movement but also the contribution from different segments (i.e. a flat back syndrome). Is the rhythm and fluidity normal for this movement.

The Spine

Extension can be an exciting part of the examination if the patient topples backwards - do not allow this to happen! Hold on to the pelvis **"lean backwards as far as you can go. I have got you, you are safe and will not fall"** (Fig 75).

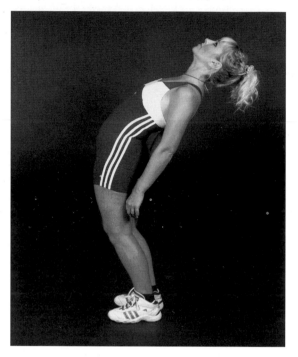

Fig. 75. Extension of the lumbar segment is about 40°.

Lateral flexion **"Slide your left hand down the outside of your left leg"**.
Again this can be measured as hand to mid thigh, knee etc. (Fig 76).

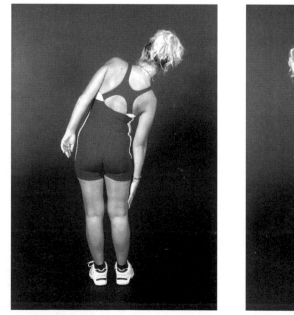 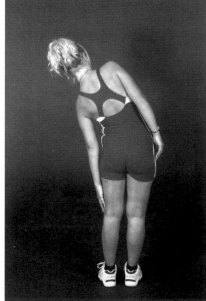

Fig. 76.. Lateral flexion.

The Spine

Neurology.

Tone.
Muscle resting tone is often the first and most vital clue as it can suggest a central or peripheral lesion. Increase in tone suggests an upper motor neurone pathology.

Power

Root value	Muscle test
L1/2	Hip flexion
L3/4	Knee extension
L4/5	Ankle dorsiflexion
L5	Long toe extensor
S1/2	Ankle plantar flexion

Reflexes.
This includes checking the superficial reflexes, deep tendon jerks and the plantar response. Remember that in cord compression the superficial reflexes below the level of the compression will be lost (except the plantar reflex which is altered) and the deep reflexes will be exaggerated.

Superficial reflex	Root value	Technique
Abdominal reflex	T10	Stroke gently from lateral to medial the four quadrants of the abdominal wall around the umbilicus and observe for symmetry of muscle contraction
Cremasteric	L1/2	Stroke the medial thigh lightly and watch for contaction of the scrotal skin

Deep Reflexes

Root value	Reflex
L3/4	Knee jerk
S1	Ankle jerk

The Spine

There are several ways of eliciting reflexes. **The knee reflex** can be adequately demonstrated by holding the thigh and taking most of the weight of the leg. Ask the patient to relax, establish the site of the patellar tendon and use the hammer provided. Alternately sit the patient on the edge of a bed with the legs hanging Freely and tap the patella tendon.

Ankle jerks can be tested with the patient sat on the edge of the bed with the ankle free, or lying on the couch prone with the feet over the edge.
Remember establish if the reflex is absent, reduced, normal or brisk. A very brisk reflex can be more suitably established by tapping with the finger rather than a tendon hammer. Re-enforcement techniques may be used if the reflex is depressed (see chapter on cervical spine).

Sensation.

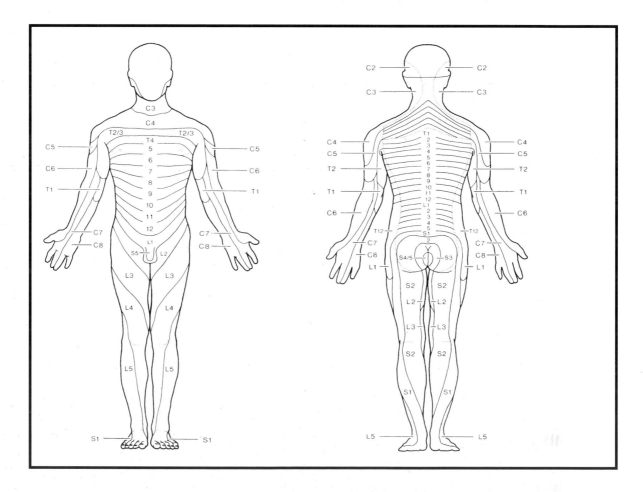

Sensation can be rapidly assessed by gentle stroking of the skin, and asking the patient to compare sides. Be clear in testing individual dermatomes of any area that is different. Establish is this hyper or hypoaesthetic. Cotton wool and sterile pinprick can further define decreased sensation but be gentle. Remember the introductory story! It is unlikely that in the exam you will be expected to demonstrate the cremesteric or bulbocavernosus reflexes, but you should know about the importance of these tests and their diagnostic implications.

Power

Check individual myotomes in the lower limbs.
(See Fig's 80-91)

Root level	Muscle test
L1-2	Flexion of hip
L3	Extension of knee
L4	Dorsiflexion of ankle
L5	Extension of hallux
S1	Plantarflexion of ankle
S2	Flexion of knee

Specific tests

These are provocative manoeuvers to elicit irritation of nerve roots. Always begin with the normal side first so that the patient is aware of what the test involves. Be gentle!

Femoral Stretch.

Lay the patient prone and extend the hip to a comfortable degree. Then flex the knee. A positive test is when the patient comments that there is a sudden increase in pain in the anterior thigh descending to the knee.
Do not be fooled by false positive tests where simple stretching of the quads is misinterpreted as pain. The femoral nerve arises from roots L 2,3,4. (Fig 77)

FABER manoeuvre.

This stands for Flexion, ABduction, External Rotation of the hip to adopt the "Cobbler" position or the position for testing sartorius.
By pressing down on the knee, pain in the back indicates sacroiliac problems, pain in the hip a hip problem.

Sciatic Stretch

These tests for root tension signs are performed with the patient supine on the couch.

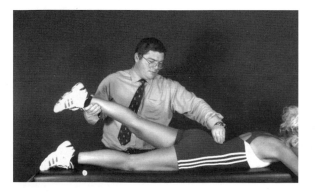

Fig. 77. Reverse straight leg raise or femoral stretch test. Resultant pain raises suspicion about the Femoral nerve and L4 root.

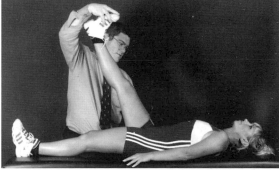

Fig. 78. Lesegue's Test. Increasing the sciatic stretch by dorsiflexion of the ankle.

The Spine

The Straight Leg Raise (SLR) is performed by gently lifting the leg with the ankle relaxed and the knee extended. Most people can get to 90 degrees quite comfortably but age and concurrent hip disease can limit this.

Remember not to push too far in the patient with a THR, as dislocation will not gain you extra points.

A positive test occurs if the patient has pain developing early on in the manoeuvre in the territory of the sciatic nerve. A straight leg raise of less than 60 degrees with pain in the appropriate distribution suggests nerve root irritation. Again beware of a false positive test where the pain is only felt in the lumbar spine or there is limitation as a result of hamstring tightness. Again always begin with the normal side. *A cross- positive straight leg raise* occurs when the patient complains of pain on the involved side during elevation of the normal leg. This is pathognomonic of nerve root compression.

Lasegue's Test.

This is an extension of the SLR where dorsiflexion of the ankle intensifies the pain the patient reports on SLR. (Fig 78)

Bowstring Test.

During the SLR, as you reach the pain point, flex the knee 15 degrees and this should dramatically reduce the pain. Rest the patient's leg in this position on your shoulder and then firmly compress the sciatic nerve in the popliteal fossa. This again stretches the peroneal nerve and should recreate the pain. (Fig 79)

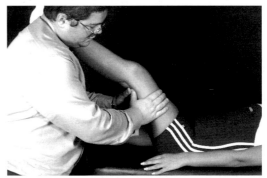

Fig. 79. Bowstring Test. Peroneal stretch is recreated by digital pressure.

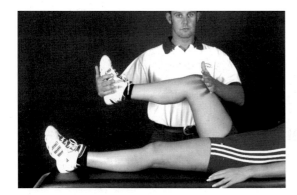

*Fig.80. Testing Iliopsoas (Femoral nerve; **L1, L2, L3**). The hip is resisted in flexion with the knee flexed.*

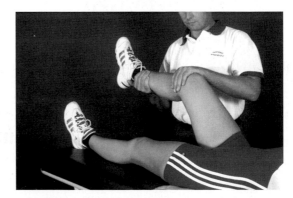

*Fig.81. Testing Quadriceps Femoris (Femoral nerve; L2, **L3, L4**). Extending the leg against resistance with the hip and knee flexed.*

The Spine

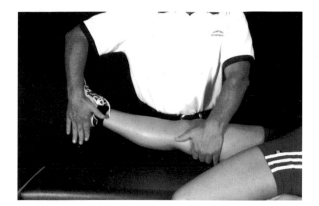

Fig.82. Adductors (Obturator nerve; **L2, L3**, L4).

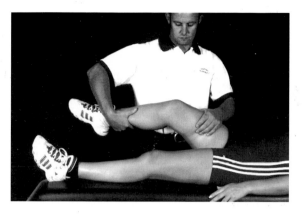

Fig.83. Gluteus Medius and Minimus (Superior Gluteal nerve; **L4, L5**, S1). Resisted internal rotation of the hip when it and the knee are both flexed.

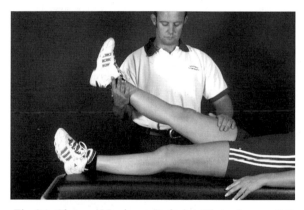

Fig.84. Gluteus Maximus (Inferior Gluteal nerve; **L5, S1**, S2). Resisted extension of the hip.

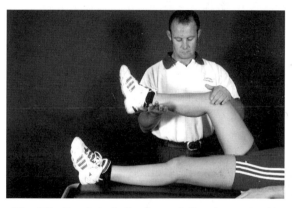

Fig.85. Resisted flexion of the knee testing semitendinosus, semimembranosus and biceps (L5, **S1** and S2).

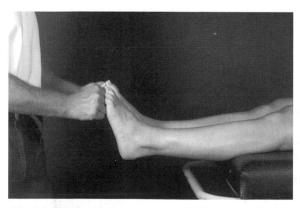

Fig.86. Testing gastrocnemius (Tibial nerve; S1, S2). Resisted plantar flexion of the ankle. A quick screening test at the beginning of the examination is to ask the patient to stand on tiptoes initially both feet together then individually. Always test this muscle specifically, if a problem is found in the screen as age, balance proprioception may confuse the issue.

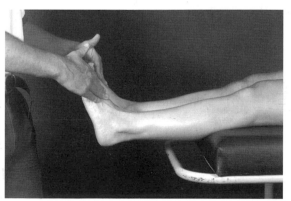

Fig.87. Testing Tibialis Anterior (Deep Peroneal nerve; **L4**, L5). Resisted dorsiflexion of the ankle.

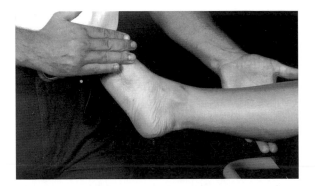

Fig.88. Testing Tibialis Posterior (Tibial nerve; L4, L5). Resisted inversion of the foot, an important specific muscle test, especially in the rheumatoid foot and ankle exam (see later).

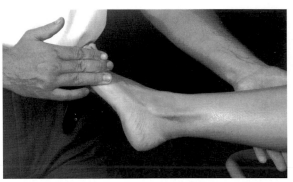

Fig.89. Testing Peroneus Longus and Brevis (Superficial Peroneal nerve; L5, S1). Resisted evertion of the foot.

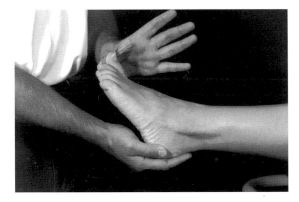

Fig.90. Testing Flexor Hallux Longus (Tibial nerve; L5, **S1, S2**). Resisted flexion of the terminal phalanx of great toe.

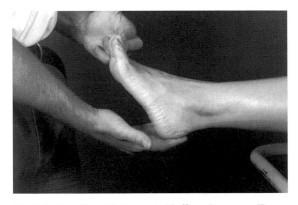

Fig.91. Testing Extensor Hallux Longus (Deep Peroneal nerve; **L5**, S1). Resisted extension of the terminal phalanx of great toe.

Finish the examination by a quick look of hips and confirm adequacy of peripheral pulses by examing the dorsalis pedis or posterior tibial pulses.

The Hip

Mr Andrew Roberts FRCS, DM
Consultant Orthopaedic Surgeon

EXPOSURE

Walking aids, external appliances and footwear.

LOOK

From the front *(stand patient facing you)*

Deformity	knee & feet
Skin	scars and circulatory disturbances.
Contour	
Wasting	

From side *(turn affected side toward you)*

Deformity	flexion attitude and lumbar lordosis.
Skin	

From behind

Deformity Lumbar spine
Buttocks
Popliteal creases

> **Pelvis Position**
> Pelvis level with symmetrical stance
> Pelvis not level with symmetrical stance
> Pelvis level with asymmetrical stance
> Pelvis not level with asymmetrical stance

From front

Pelvic tilt (check levels of ASIS; stance symmetrical; check ankle and knee)
Ask for blocks
Trendelenberg

Gait

Walk away and towards

> **Gait**
> Short Leg
> Trendelenberg
> Rigid
> Antalgic
> Weak
> Supratentorial

The Hip

SUPINE ON COUCH

 Leg Length   See special tests

 Feel   Along line of inguinal ligament

         Posterior greater trochanter

 Move   Thomas test

         Flexion / extension

         Rotation in flexion

         Abduction / adduction in extension

LATERAL ON COUCH (LIE WITH AFFECTED SIDE UP)

 Abductor power

PRONE ON COUCH (CARE IF FFD OR IN PAIN)

 Gluteal bulk

 Rotation in extension

ADJACENT JOINT

 Lumbar spine

 Knee

CLINICAL CASES

 Osteoarthritis

 Avascular necrosis

 Post joint replacement

The Hip

EXPOSURE

Again remember to expose properly, classically this is from chest downwards, but you must respect the patient's modesty - be guided by the examiner. Use this initial few seconds to take in the scene. A mother with a child on her knee, wheelchair in the corner, pensioner with crutches propped up against a chair or a young "biker" with a below knee prosthesis under the couch. Get your mind working so that you can focus on the positive clinical findings.

INSPECTION

From the front
Stand with the patient facing you. Be prepared that they may not be able to stand unaided, be ready to support the patient, this alone tells you a lot about the patient and tells a lot to the examiner about how you undertake your clinical practice.

Deformity
Look at the knee. It may be in valgus or varus; a fixed flexion deformity maybe evident.

Skin
Comment on scars from previous accidents or surgery. Why would a young adult have a well-healed scar from an anterior approach to the hip? Sinus scars may give you further information. Circulatory disturbances show as hair loss or trophic changes in the skin.

Contour and Wasting
Note any quadriceps wasting.

From side
Turn the affected side towards you and repeat the routine.

Deformity
The flexion attitude and lumbar lordosis can be assessed. Is the patient compensating for a fixed flexion contracture by excessive lordosis? This is certainly worth commenting about.

Skin
Are other scars now visible?

From behind

Deformity
Look at the lumbar spine and comment on alignment. A degenerative scoliosis may mean that the "hip" pain is originating from the spine, or hip adduction may have caused a lumbar scoliosis.

Wasting
Look at the buttocks. In the thinner patient gluteal wasting is an important physical finding. Remember to look for sinuses - this may indicate an old TB hip that has been enrolled for the exam.

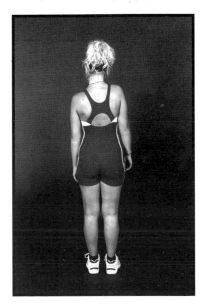

Fig. 87 Inspection from behind. Not only can you start to focus on muscle wasting, scars, pelvic obliquity but look to see if weight distribution is even on both legs.

The Hip

From front

Assess the pelvic tilt, check the levels of anterior superior iliac spines, is the stance symmetrical? Look at the distance between the knees and ankles.

Ask for blocks and level the pelvis. Ask the patient when they feel they are level. This is a rapid and accurate method of assessing shortening.

The Trendelenberg test is very important and one that you must be able to demonstrate and feel at "home" with. There are many methods described, one way that rather slickly shows any problem is to face the patient and ask them to rest their hands on yours held in front of you. Then ask them to stand on their bad leg. This produces a drop from the horizontal plane of the pelvis but also increased pressure on your hand on the affected side. Be clear why a test is positive, as it will guide your remaining examination. A positive test can be due to hip abductors that are failing, pain, a biomechanical disadvantage (long established CDH or gross Coxa vara) or paralysis (old polio or post THR exposure).

Gait

Ask the patient to walk away and then back towards you. It is essential to recognise the differences between a Trendelenberg, an antalgic or a short leg gait. Consider each aspect of the gait cycle. The stance phase during walking accounts for 65% of the whole cycle, the rhythm is important, in particular the toe-off, swing and heel strike. Look for pelvic obliquity.

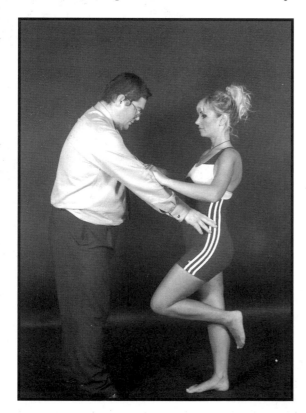

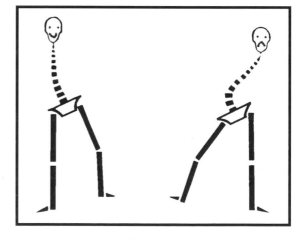

Fig. 88 The Trendelenberg Test. Look for the more obvious drop in the patient's shoulder in the gross case, feel the pressure changes on your hands in the more subtle case or ask the patient to maintain the position for a short while to see the fatigue positive case.

The Hip

Supine on Couch

Leg Length

There are many ways to demonstrate shortening. We have found the following method to be useful.

Examination begins as the patient walks towards you or stands in front. If you are introduced and they are already on the couch, ensure you stand close to them and make a comment about obvious visible limb length discrepancy.

Adjust their position on the couch even if they are straight - already demonstrating that you are checking. If there is significant shortening then one heel will be above the other.

Assess the over limb length, apparent length can be measured from the umbilicus or xiphisternum (exposure is so important) to the medial malleolus of each limb.

True or actual leg length is from the anterior superior iliac spine to the medial malleolus. The problem arises when the patient has an adduction or abduction deformity. In this case, place the good

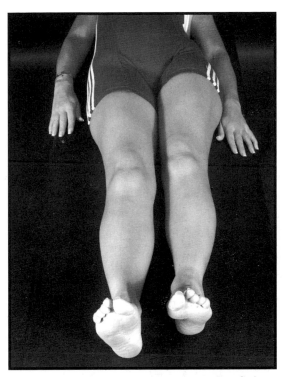

Fig.91 Leg length discrepancy may be obvious, but check the pelvis is level.

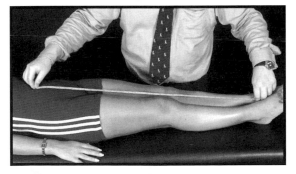

Fig.89 Apparent leg length is only useful when compared to actual leg length.

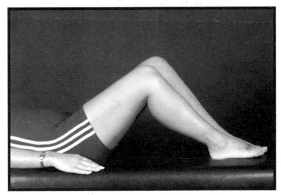

Fig.92 Ask yourself where is the discrepancy; tibia or femur and if it is the femur above or below the greater trochanter?

limb in the same degree of deformity and perform the measurements.

We have mentioned the use of blocks previously and they can be a useful adjunct in this type of case.

Flex the knees up now and place the heels together. This shows whether the shortening is in the femur or tibia (Galeazzi test). The bone lengths can be measured but this is not particularly accurate.

Palpate

Along line of inguinal ligament and posterior greater trochanter.

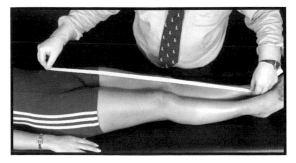

Fig.90 Actual leg length, measure carefully from the anterior superior iliac spine to the medial malleolus. A more accurate method that may be brought up in a discussion is either a scanogram or spiral CT scout film.

The Hip

Move

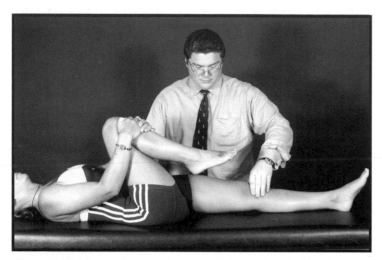

Fig.93 Thomas's Test. Again an absolute need to be at home with the test. Demonstrate you have eliminated the lumbar lordosis with your free hand.

Thomas Test - again another test that you must be able to demonstrate smoothly.
MUST STABILISE PELVIS WHEN TESTING FLEXION

Flex the affected hip as far as it will go (comment on the range of flexion). Place your hand behind the small of the patient's back.

Ask and help them to flex up the non-affected side. This obliterates the lumbar lordosis, ***check.***

Now ask the patient to extend the affected side. A fixed flexion deformity will become apparent (comment on the degree).

This can then be repeated on the other side. The normal range of flexion is about 120°.

Now assess internal and external rotation with the hip and knee flexed at 90°.

Hold the knee with one hand and the foot with the other.

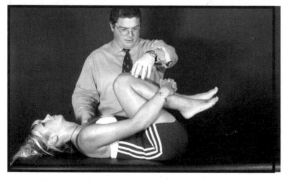

Fig.94 Flexion of the hip.

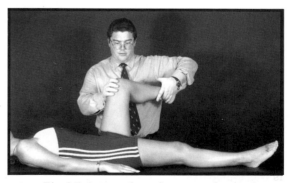

Fig.95 Internal and external rotation can be tested with the hip flexed to 90°.

The leg can then be rested on the couch and rolled into internal and external rotation to assess rotation in extension, this may be better performed with the patient prone.

The Hip

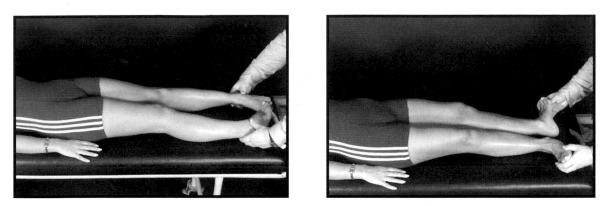

Fig.96 Then assess with the hip extended to neutral. Is there a difference?

Assess not only the range of movement but stiffness, discomfort and muscle tone. Take care not to hurt the patient.

Abduction can sometimes be difficult to quantify due to pelvic and lumbar spine movement. There are two ways to avoid this problem. If the pelvis is palpated during abduction and adduction, any movement signifies the end of the range of movement in the hip. This may be the best way to proceed as the examiner can see you are ensuring that the movements are in the hip.

Another method is to measure abduction in the good limb first.

Abduct the normal whilst palpating the anterior superior iliac spine and leave the leg over the edge of the couch. Now abduct the abnormal leg. The normal leg will steady the pelvis. The normal range is 40°.

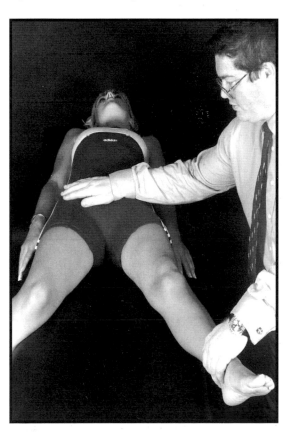

Fig.97 Measuring Abduction. Make a show of feeling where the ASIS are, fix them with your forearm and assess the arc of movement up to the point where the pelvis begins to rotate.

The Hip

Moving the examining leg over the good side by flexing the hip slightly assesses adduction. Normal range about 30°.

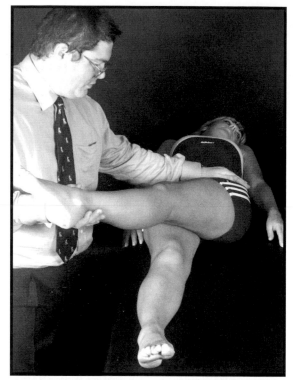

Fig. 98 Measuring Adduction. Again stabilise the pelvis and assess hip motion before pelvic movement can be felt.

Lateral on Couch *(Lie with affected side up)*

Ask the patient to abduct the leg against resistance whilst palpating the gluteal muscles. You can use the MRC scale of muscle power here quite elegantly to demonstrate support of a positive Trendelenberg Test. This is very important in patients who have had previous surgery to ensure good abductor power.

Prone on Couch *(CARE if FFD or in pain)*

Gluteal bulk can further be defined. The normal range of extension is really quite variable but a maximum of about 20°
is normal. Again take the opportunity to palpate and grade extensor power as well as range of movement.

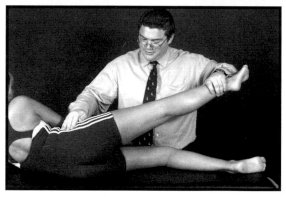

Fig. 99 Abducting the hip against gravity and then resistance allows the Gluteal function to be assessed.

Rotation in extension does allow a convenient and clear demonstration of restricted movement. The knee is flexed up to 90° and feet held apart to demonstrate a normal range of 35° internal rotation, and crossed over to demonstrate external rotation of about 45°.

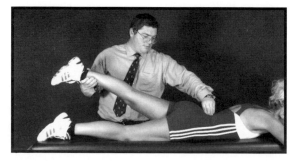

Fig. 100 Extension of the hip.

The Hip

Remember to stabilise the pelvis with your hand or forearm during this manoeuvre to ensure that any movement detected is not due to pelvic rock.

Look for any asymmetry as this may indicate malrotation of one limb or movement excessively in internal or external rotation thus indicating a bilateral rotational abnormality such as persistent femoral anteversion. The femoral neck anteversion can be formally tested whilst the patient is prone.

Adjacent Joint

Always examine the lumbar spine and knees.

Special Tests

The unsound arthrodesis *(spasm of muscles)*

Not such a rare case in the exam as there are several patients with old TB of the hip.

If the good leg is flexed up and the patient holds their knee, use one hand to palpate the lesser trochanter and ilio-psoas, then with the other hand smartly abduct the arthrodesed leg.

If there is a protective contraction of the muscle group, then the arthrodesis is not sound.

Telescoping of hip

This may help alert suspicion to laxity of the surrounding soft tissues following total hip replacement, at the extreme frank pistoning of a femoral component.

Problem:

Fixed knee flexion:

-Move the patient to the end of the couch to check hip extension in full.

Fixed adduction at the hip on one side:

-Place the other hip in a matching position by crossing the legs.
Then proceed to measure legs.

The Knee

Mr Simon Roberts MA, FRCS (Orth), FFSEM.
Consultant Sports Injury Surgeon

EXPOSURE

INSPECTION

Walking / mobility aids; external appliances.

From the front

Deformity knee alignment
patellar rotation
foot rotation

Think about the "Q" Angle
Skin
Contours
Wasting

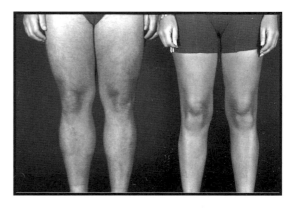

Fig. 101 The anterior view of the knee allows you to pick up early signs of wasting, effusion, deformity and surgery.

From the side

Deformity knee attitude (flexion or recurvatum), foot (equinus)
Skin
Contours swelling

From behind

Deformity hindfoot, physiological valgus
Skin popliteal swelling, wasting hamstrings and calf

Gait

Limb Length pelvic obliquity
Walk Away antalgic, lateral thrust, stiff knee, back knee, short leg
Walk Towards

The Knee

Supine on the Couch

Laying flat	**Inspection**	***Quads bulk and circumference***
Palpation		Effusion (wipe, balottment, patellar tap)
		Tenderness
Movement		Active extension (quadriceps lag)
		Passive extension (FFD, recurvatum)
		Active flexion
		Passive flexion
		Feel for crepitus and meniscal cyst
At 80 degrees	**Palpation**	Extensor mechanism
(sit on foot)		Patellar tendon
		Tibial tuberosity
		Inferior pole of patellar
		Medial joint line
		Lateral joint line
		MCL & LCL (origin, tendon & insertion)
Knee flexed	Posterior Cruciate	Posterior sag/quads active test.

Knee 20 degrees flexion Valgus & varus stress Abnormal movement
Opening of joint
Correction of deformity
End-point (grade I, II, III)
Patellar facets lateral and
medial femoral condyles
Lachmann's

Knee at 20 degrees with legs crossed over

	Palpate	Size
		Tenderness -medial and lateral facets
		Patellar grind
		Clarke's test
Provocative test		Meniscus, McMurray
		Pivot shift.
Prone dial test		Posteriorlateral corner
		Foot/thigh
		Epicondyler axis

The Knee

Non-Mechanical Tests

Pulses
Neurology
Joint above and below

Special Cases

Patello-femoral Q angle and tracking
                     Apprehension
                     Femoral anteversion & tibial torsion
Anterior instability
Posterior instability

6 Point summary

1. **Look - Standing/walking**

2. **Look/Feel - supine - extended.**

3. **Move/Feel - Flexed 80 degrees (PCL).**

4. **Special tests - One test each for ACL, MCL, LCL and Posterolateral corner. Provocative meniscus.**

5. **Patella.**

6. **General.**

The Knee

INTRODUCTION

As with all other sections, the examination described here tries to cover most pathologies with which you will be presented. However, although superficially it may seem impressive to know and to demonstrate three tests of ACL (Anterior Cruciate Ligament) insufficiency, it could be misconstrued as not understanding, or recognising, the positive result from the first test, just one Lachmans.

Adapt your examination not only to the type of case (young male athlete versus elderly post Total Knee Replacement female) but also to the findings you are able to demonstrate.

EXPOSURE

Remember to expose properly, trousers not only down but also out (of the equation), or skirt off. Tempting as it might be to just "roll up a trouser leg" this is seen as inadequate exposure. Again, though, judge the situation and know the time constraints of your case. In a short case "ready prepared" you will not score points or use your time usefully in this manner. Use the escape phrase "in my normal clinical practice I would expose the whole of the lower limb but ......"

INSPECTION

This involves not only looking at the patient!

Often as a subtle guide a kind patient or even examiner will leave a stick or caliper at the side of the bed to help guide your thoughts.

Do you know the difference between the different calipers available?

What is the clinical significance of a Donjoy brace?

Does a walking stick with a moulded grip give you a clue about other pathology or patient ability as compared to an ordinary cane?

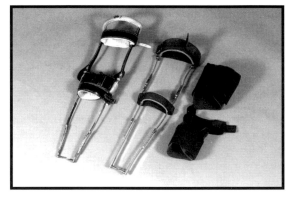

Fig.102 A knowledge of the different types and purposes of braces is important.

Why might a patient use elbow crutches as compared to axillary bearing ones?

Shoes can suggest many things with regards to limb length inequality, neurological problems or even occupation.

All these questions need to be answered in your mind before you even enter an exam.

Chat to the orthotics technicians or the physiotherapy team to clarify the orthoses in your mind as an understanding here can set you off on a flying start.

The Knee

FROM THE FRONT

Deformity
Knee valgus/varus alignment, patellar rotation and foot rotation are important clinical signs.

Skin
So what are the incisions around the knee and how do they give clues?

Open menisectomy, high tibial osteotomy, arthroscopy, lateral release all give clues about the pathology.

Did the wound not heal well?

Is there evidence of healing by second intention or a persistent sinus?

Were things bad enough to require a split skin graft or even a local rotational flap?

Is this a major trauma with a bulky free flap whose pedicle may affect the site of your proposed surgical exposure?

Do not miss faded arthroscopy portal scars.

Contours
In the athlete, the contours of the musculature of the thigh are evident but, in the obese, these are hidden.

Wasting
This can be either global or local.

Wasting can be acute following disuse from recent plaster confinement or pain inhibition, or long term from neurogenic causes such as old polio.

Comment on any swellings or lumps.

FROM THE SIDE

Deformity
Look at the attitude of the knee - is it held in flexion or recurvatum?

Remember if you find these deformities, you want at the end of the examination to be able to say they are fixed, partially correctable or wholly correctable.

Comment on any foot equinus as this can affect the knee posture.

Is there a patellar sag or a prominent tibial tubercle of an old Osgood-Slatters disease?

Skin and Countours
Comment on any significant findings.

The Knee

FROM BEHIND

Deformity
Look at the hindfoot - this can result in a physiological valgus.
Does it correct with tip toe standing ?
Large varicose veins or a popiteal aneurysm will affect your surgical options.

Is there a Baker's cyst or a silhouetted lateral meniscal cyst?

Skin and Contours
Comment on any scars not previously noted.

Wasting
Look for wasting of the hamstrings and calf muscles.

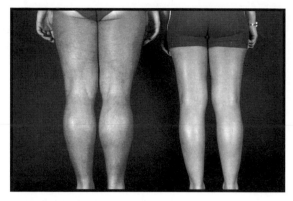

Fig. 103 The posterior view of the knee continues your inspection. Is there an obvious Baker's cyst or popliteal aneurysm?

The Knee

Gait

Never forget that assessment of function is vital and may illustrate not only the problem in the knee but highlight your attention to other complicating factors that may affect your management.

Ask the patient to walk away and walk towards you.

The varus thrust of a knee is an important clinical finding.

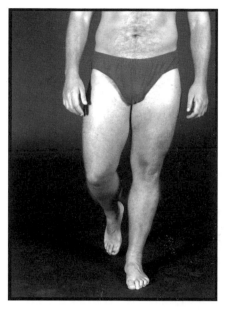

Fig. 104 Gait is vital in the assessment of the knee. Ask the patient to walk with and without shoes and if possible with and without their walking aids. Break the gait cycle up in your mind into its component parts. Learn to recognise the pattern of different gaits.

Does the varus / valgus deformity worsen?

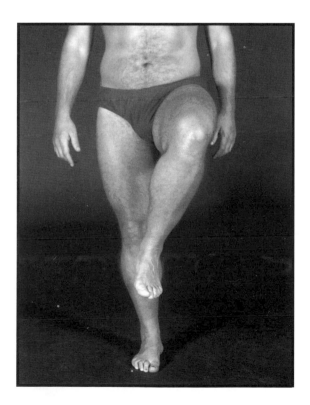

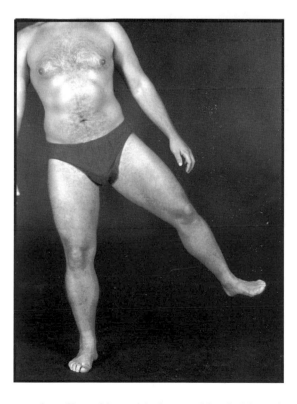

Fig. 105 Hop Test. Two part functional stress test; hop on the affected leg with the good leg held out in abduction (Valgus stress on the affected knee) and with the good leg held in adduction (Varus stress on affected knee). Again one for the young sports instability patient.

A stiff knee or a knee with a fixed flexion deformity can be observed during the gait.

The Knee

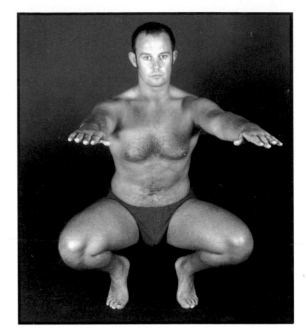

Fig.106 Functional Tests of the knee include squatting, kneeling, "duck waddling" (walking while fully squatted), stationary jogging. These tests are very appropriate for the "young sports instability patient" but should not be so vigorously applied to the "elderly revision TKR".

SUPINE ON THE COUCH

Lying flat   -   The hips should be extended to reduce hamstring tension.

Inspection
Comment on the bulk of the quadriceps, ideally the circumference at a specific point should be measured.

Assess tone. This can be demonstrated to **"Brace knee into couch"**. Lift the heel up to assess fixed flexion deformity or sag.

Limb Length
Pick up both legs by the heel. Is there fixed flexion deformity or recurvatum ?
Inequality may be obvious by the presence of pelvic obliquity but may need careful examination by comparing sides with the knee flexed when the patient is supine on the couch.

The site of shortening can be identified as femoral or tibial by careful placement of the heels and correct alignment of the pelvis.

With the knees flexed, a posterior sag of a tibia becomes more obvious. You can use a pencil to rest on the tibial tubercle to compare sides.

Palpation
Test for an effusion using the wipe test,(detect 10 ml) patellar balottment and patellar tap. (detect > 25ml)

Grade the effusion I, II or III.

Be systematic when trying to elicit the exact site of tenderness.

In knees this is often the key, is it solely medial or lateral, does it occur on pressure over the patella (perform patellofemoral tests).

Trigger points can help focus your examination.

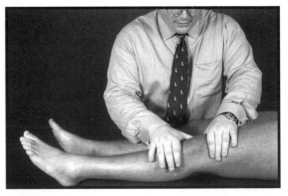

Fig.107 The Wipe Test. Milking a small effusion down from the suprapatellar pouch.

The Knee

MOVEMENT

The normal range of movement is 0°-145°.

Look for active extension and a extensor lag because of quadriceps weakness or pain inhibition by completing passive motion. (Possible due to quadriceps weakness and pain inhibition)

You must differentiate between an extensor lag and fixed flexion deformity.

Look for hyperextension by lifting both feet off the bed. >10° is abnormal.

Active flexion can be measured not only with your goniometer but also by measuring the buttock heel distance and comparing sides.

Feel for crepitus and swellings during the range of movement. A meniscal cyst may become more evident during flexion.

The Knee - Special tests

NON-MECHANICAL TESTS

Pulses

These are often forgotten in the excitement.

Look for obvious clues in the lower limb that indicate ischaemia, such as loss of hair, trophic skin changes, colour or previous toe amputations.

Remember this case may not be being used as a straight forward OA knee but to introduce topics of operative planning.

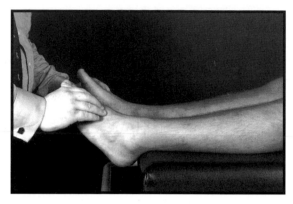

Fig.108 Do not forget to feel for peripheral pulses, a lack of which may alter your diagnosis and management plan.

Neurology

It is vital to establish the pre-operative neurology of an OA varus knee.

Look at joint above and below

The Knee - Special tests

Q-ANGLE
Technique

Ensure the limbs are at right-angles to a line joining the two anterior-superior iliac spines (ASIS).

Draw a line from the ASIS to the midpoint of the patella and from the midpoint of the tibial tubercle.

Take care to ensure that the hip and foot are in a neutral position.

Remember this is important in describing associated deformities of fixed flexion and recurvatum of the knee.

Clinical relevance
The normal Q-angle is 13° for males and 18° for females.

The test can be enhanced by assessment of the Q-angle with the knee flexed (normally 0°) or with the quadriceps flexed (normal <10°).

Look for associated chondromalacia patellae, subluxing patella, increased femoral anteversion, genu valgum, lateral displacement of tibial tubercle or increased tibial torsion.

Other related tests
A-angle
A **vertical** line divides the patella into two, a second line drawn from the tibial tubercle to the lower pole of the patella.

References
Arno S. The A-angle. A quantitative measurement of patella alignment.
J. Orthop. Sports Phys. Ther. 1990, 112:237-42.
Tria AJ, Palumbo RC. Conservative treatment of patellofemoral pain.
Semin. Orthop. 1990, 5: 115-21.

APPREHENSION (FAIRBANK'S) TEST

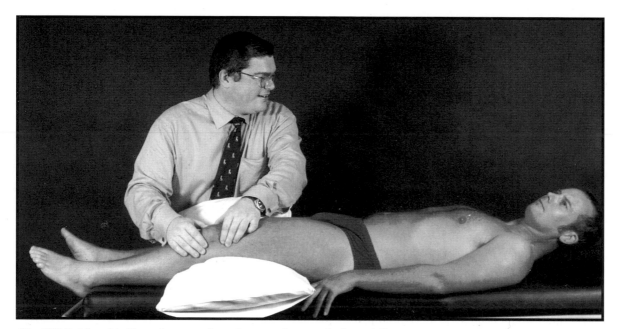

Fig. 109 Fairbank's Test. An apprehension test for patella instability. Be cautious and watch the patient's face.

Technique

With the patient supine and the quadriceps relaxed, the knee is flexed to 30° whilst lateral pressure is applied to the patella.

Clinical relevance

If the quadriceps is contracted in an attempt to realign the patella, the test is positive.

Reference

Hughston JC, Walsh WM, Puddu G. Patellar subluxation and dislocation.
Philadelphia, Saunders. 1984.

The Knee - Special tests

CLARKE'S SIGN

Technique
Clinical relevance

The patella is pressed against an extended knee. The patient is asked to tense the quadriceps. i.e. attempted SLR.

Pain behind the patella means a positive test. Other parts of the patella can be assessed by repeating the test at 30°, 60° and 90°.

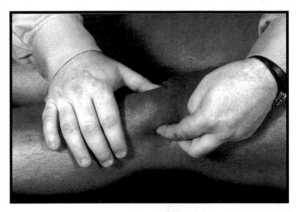

Fig.110 Assessing patella femoral joint discomfort.

Related tests

McConnell Test - the patient performs isometric quadriceps contractions at 120°, 90°, 60°, 30° and 0°. If pain is produced the test is repeated with the patella held medially. If this abolishes the pain the origin is patellofemoral.

Waldron Test - an odd test that is really common sense. Ask the patient to stand and then bend the knee to a "squat" as far as they can do safely. If anterior knee pain is reported and you can feel crepitus on movement of the patella, the test is positive for patello-femoral joint arthrtis.

Passive Patellar Tilt - the lateral border of the patella is lifted whilst still in the trochlea. A normal angle is >**5°**.

Lateral Pull Test - with the patient supine, active contraction of the quadriceps moves the patella superiorly and laterally by the same proportion. An excess lateral movement is a sign of maltracking.

Zohler's Sign - with the knee relaxed and the patella pulled distally, pain with quadriceps contraction is indicative of patellofemoral pathology.

References
McConnell J. The management of chondromalacia patellae: a long-term solution.
Aust. J. Physiother. 1986; 32:215-223.
Kolowich PA, Paulos LE, Rosenberg TD, Farnsworth S. Lateral release of the patella.
Am J. Sports Med. 1990. 18: 359-65.
Strobel M, Stedtfeld HW. Diagnostic evaluation of the knee.
Berlin, Springer. 1990.

Other tests
Femoral anteversion - discussed in detail in The Hip section
Tibial torsion - sit the patient on the edge of the couch, with the lower legs hanging free. Palpate the tibial tubercle and assess the angle subtended by the foot with the tibial tubercle.Compare both sides.
Medial and Lateral Displacement - lower legs hanging free over the edge of the couch, Grasp the patient's foot between your own knees. Use one hand to steady the distal femur and with the other hand, apply a translational force to the proximal tibia.

The Knee - Special tests

MEDIAL / LATERAL LAXITY

Valgus and varus sress tests

Technique

The examiner applies either a valgus or varus force with the knee at $0°$ and $30°$

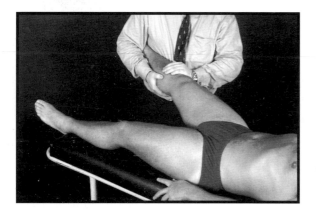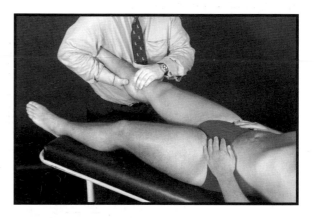

Fig.111 Valgus stress of the knee. A lax medial collateral or deficient lateral compartment? Is there an end point? When instability is found at $30°$ of flexion, injury is likely to be limited to one or a combination of the medial compartment ligaments (Tibial collateral ligament, medial collateral ligament, medial capsule). If found at $0°$ also, then suspicion about posterior structures as well is raised (Posterior capsule, Posterior Cruciate Ligament).

Fig.112 Varus stress of the knee. Is the deformity correctable or fixed? Instability at $30°$ suggests injury to lateral structures (Lateral Collateral Ligament, Iliotibial Tract, Lateral capsule). If instability also is found at $0°$ then consider further injury to biceps tendon, arcuatepopliteus complex, popliteofibular ligament, ACL and PCL

Clinical significance

A positive finding in extension is seen with multiple/complex ligament injuries.

This has been graded as:-

      I   (0 to 5mm),
      II   (5 to 10mm) or
      III   (>10mm).

A pure medial or lateral complex injury is indicated when the test is positive only at $30°$.

A positive test in extension is ALWAYS positive at $30°$ so perform in flexion first. If it is normal, then it need not be repeated in extension.

The Knee - Special tests

ANTERIOR LAXITY

Lachmann Test

Technique
With the patient supine, the knee is held at 30°.

The femur is stabilised by one hand whilst the tibia is moved forward with the other hand (in a position of slight lateral rotation).

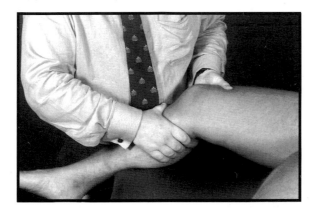

Fig. 113 Lachman Test. The ACL test. Grade I (5mm of displacement), II (5-10 mm) and III (>10mm).

Clinical significance
The test is considered positive if there is no solid end-point as indicated by injury to the anterior cruciate ligament. This can be graded as I, II or III. The clinical significance of this test is that it is the preferred assessment of the ACL. It is however, imperative that you compare sides before commenting on ACL insufficiency.

Other related tests

Position the patient with the knee over the edge of the examining table
The knee rests on the examiner's knee
The calf is stabilised between the examiner's chest and arm
Prone Lachmann (Feagin)

The Knee - Special tests

ANTERIOR DRAWER SIGN

This test is not favoured by all examiners as interpretation of the test can be difficult, i.e. is it a posterially subluxed tibia you are reducing anterially or is it a reduced tibia you are subluxing anterially?

CARE IS NEEDED.

Technique

With the knee flexed to 90° the foot is stabilised under the examiners thigh. The examiners hands are placed around the tibia (ensure the hamstrings are relaxed) and the tibia pulled forward.

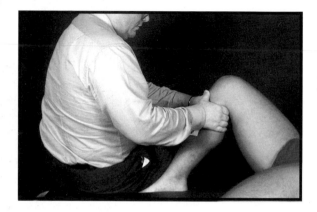

Fig. 114 Anterior Draw Sign. Not a favourite among many examiners due to difficulty in interpretation.

Clinical significance

The test is considered positive if there is more than 6mm of movement (the posterior sag test must be proven to be negative).

A negative test is found if the ACL alone is ruptured or if the drawer is blocked by a meniscal tear, haemarthrosis or muscle spasm.

Modifications

With the patient relaxed and the knee and hip flexed to 90° the tibia is grasped with both hands and the leg lifted.

By examining the drawer with the leg over the end of the bed the effect of gravity is negated and any posterior sag elimanated.

References
Butler DL, Noyes FR, Grood ES. Ligamentous restraints to anterior-posterior drawer in the human knee.
J. Bone Joint Surg. 1980 62-A: 259-270.
Weatherwax RJ. Anterior drawer sign.
Clin. Orthop. 1981, 154: 318-9

The Knee - Special tests

PIVOT SHIFT TEST

Technique
With the patient supine and the hip slightly flexed, one hand holds the foot in **internal** rotation whilst the other is placed at the knee. The knee is flexed whilst applying valgus strain.

Our preferred method, though, is to grasp the patient's foot in your axilla and to use both of your hands to control the proximal tibia.

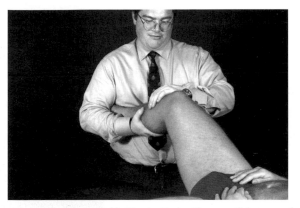

Fig. 115 Pivot Shift Test. Gain the confidence of the patient, start with small initial movements and build up to the full range of the test.

Clinical significance
The reduction of the tibia on the femur at 30° is felt as a 'clunk' in anterior cruciate deficient knees.

Modifications

Jerk Test of Hughston - is similar to the pivot shift but the hip is flexed further to 45° and the knee starts in flexion and then extended. The jerk of subluxation is felt.

Noyes Flexion-Rotation Test - the foot is held between the chest and arm with the hands supporting the tibia. The knee is flexed at 20° and a posterior movement reduces the subluxation of the tibia.

Losee Sloum

Other Tests

Jakob (Reverse Pivot Shift) - with the patient supine and relaxed the leg is supported on the examiners pelvis. The knee is flexed to 80° and the foot **externally** rotated. A positive test is indicates posterolateral instability as the tibia subluxes posteriorly.

References
Galway HR, MacIntosh DL. The lateral pivot shift: a symptom and sign of anterior cruciate ligament insufficiency.
Clin. Orthop. 1980, 147: 45-50.
Hughston JC, Noyes FR, Butler ES, Grood ES. Clinical paradoxes of anterior cruciate instability and a new test to detect its instabilty.
Orthop. Trans. 1978, 2:36.
Jakob RP, Hassler H, Staeubli HU. Observations on rotatory instability of the lateral compartment of the knee.
Acta Orthop. Scand. 1981 (Supp 191) 52: 1-32.
Liorzou. G. Knee ligaments: clinical examination. Berlin: Springer, 1991.

The Knee - Special tests

POSTERIOR LAXITY

Posterior Sag Sign

Technique
With the flexed at 90° the position of the tibia is noted.

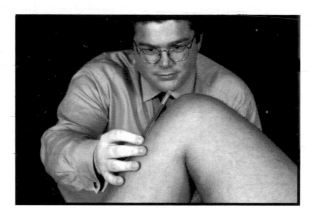

Fig. 116 Posterior Sag Sign. A positive sign can be excentuated by placing a pen on the tibial tubercle but beware of the unilateral Osgood Schlatters.

Clinical significance
A positive sign is noted if the tibia 'sags' and is indicative of posterior laxity (compare to the other side while viewing across the knees).

Other related tests

Hughston's Test - is performed in the same position. The foot is slightly internally rotated and posterior force applied. A movement posteriorly indicates posteromedial laxity. This is repeated in external rotation to indicate posterolateral laxity.

Quadriceps active test - If there is a posterior sag, it may be reduced by quadriceps contraction with the knee flexed to 90 degrees and the foot fixed.

Quadriceps neutral point - The patella tendon runs distally and anteriorly near extension and distally and posteriorly in deep flexion in the normal knee. At about 80 degrees of flexion it runs distally perpendicular to the tibial plateau and therefore has no saggital plane component.

References
Hughston JC, Norwood LA. The posterolateral drawer test and external rotational recurvatum test for posterolateral rotatory instability of the knee.
Clin. Orthop. 1980; 147: 83

The Knee - Special tests

TESTS FOR MENISCAL INJURY

MCMURRAY TEST

Technique
With the knee flexed internal rotation is applied and the knee is extended testing the lateral meniscus.

This is repeated in external rotation to test the medial meniscus.

Clinical implications
A torn meniscus produces a click accompanied by pain.

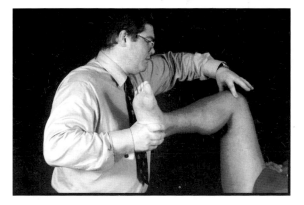

Fig.117 McMurray Test. The workhorse of meniscal testing.

Other related tests

Apley's Grind Test - is performed with the patient prone. Rotation is aplied as above but alternating compression and distraction helps to distinguish a meniscal (painful on compression) or ligamentous lesion (painful on distraction).

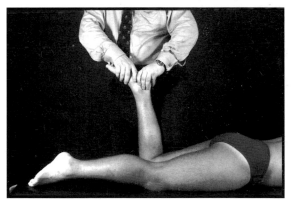

Fig.118 Apley Grind Test. Very useful for differentiating between meniscal and ligamentous injury.

Helferts Test - relies on the relationship of the tibial tuberosity to the patella. When the knee is flexed these line up, as the knee is extended the tubercle should line up with the lateral border of the patella. A meniscal tear will block this normal movement.

References
McMurray TP. The semilunar cartilages.
Br. J. Surg. 1942. 29: 407-414.
Apley AG. The diagnosis of meniscus injuries. Some new clinical methods.
J. Bone Joint Surg. 1947; 29-B: 78-84.
Helfet A. Disorders of the knee.
Philadelphia. Lippincott ., 1974.

The Knee - Special tests

PLICA TESTS

Technique
The knee is flexed to 30° and the patella is moved medially.

Clinical implications
Pain is caused as a medial plica is trapped between the femur and patella.

Other tests
Stutter Test - The knee is brought from flexion to extension actively whilst the examiner palpates the patella. A plica will cause the patella to stutter between 60° and 45°.

Hughston's Plica Test - The foot and tibia are held in internal rotation and the patella pushed medially. A 'popping' is felt medially if a plica is present on passive flexion and extension.

References
Mital MA, Hayden I. Pain in the knee in children: the medial plica shelf syndrome. *Orthop. Clin. North Am. 1979; 10: 713-22*

The Knee - Special tests

TESTS FOR KNEE SWELLING

BULGE TEST (WIPE) STROKING TEST

Technique
The medial joint is emptied by stroking from distal to proximal. The fluid is then pushed from the lateral side by a reverse motion.

Clinical implications
The fluid is seen passing from the one side to the other. This can pick up as little as 5ml of extra fluid within the knee.

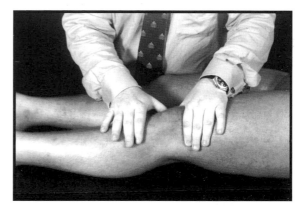

Fig.119 Bulge Test. Having milked the effusion from the suprapatellar pouch the fluid can be displaced medially and laterally by gentle pressure. An effusion can be further demonstrated by including the Patella Tap Test in your examination.

Modifications
Indentation test relies on excess fluid filling the normal lateral indentation when the knee is flexed. The sooner this occurs the greater the fluid in the knee.

Other tests

Fluctuation test
is performed by pressing the fluid from the suprapatellar pouch to the oppposite side of the joint.

Patellar tap
signifies a large effusion. The floating patella is knocked against the femur. This can be performed after the suprapatellar pouch is emptied.

References
Mann G, Finsterbush A, Frankel U, Maton Y. A method of diagnosing small amounts of fluid in the knee.
J. Bone Joint Surg. 1991; 73: 346-7.

The Foot and Ankle

Mr. Nilesh K.Makwana. FRCS (Ed.& Glas.)FRCS (Orth)
Consultant Orthopaedic Surgeon

Mr. Patrick W.Laing. FRCS   Mr. Simon O. Hill. FRCS, FRCS (Orth)
Consultant Orthopaedic Surgeons

Mr Paul Cool. FRCS (Orth) Mr. W.J. Hart. FRCS, FRCS (Orth)
Consultant Orthopaedic Surgeons

The foot and ankle are part of the locomotor system and are intricately linked to the other components. Failure in one can affect the function of another e.g. Tibialis posterior dysfunction can affect gait and lead to back pain, knee pain and hip pain. Spinal problems may affect the neuromuscular function of the foot directly or referred pain may be the reason why the patient has presented to a foot and ankle surgeon. Central to understanding why things can go wrong is the understanding of the biomechanics and function of the foot and ankle. Knowing the biomechanics and gait with a clear history, examination and appropriate investigations, the patterns of foot and ankle dysfunction can be worked out.

Exposure

Expose the whole lower limb above the knee. Before exposing the patient it is better to observe their gait with their shoes on and using any aids It is important to have an adequate walk way to observe the patient walking at their normal velocity. Once they have been observed in normal shoes then expose them above the knee. Look for walking aids, crutches and inspect their shoes. Inspect both the outside of the shoe for rockers (forefoot, midfoot or entire sole), steel plates and the inside for orthotics. Inspect and comment on the wear patterns on the outside. Varus hindfoot will have lateral wear patterns, and planovagus feet will have medial wear. In females particularly check to see if the shoe is the right size, most are one size below. Do not forget to look at the hands, mouth and eyes for features of systemic disease like rheumatoid arthritis, psoriasis, Reiter's or even intrinsic wasting with hereditary sensory and motor neuropathy.

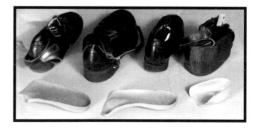

Fig. 120 Look at the footwear, what is the wear pattern, how have they been adapted, is the adaptation for deformity or muscle weakness?

Gait Patterns
Antalgic
Foot drop
Diplegic, hemiplegic
Short leg
In/ Out toeing
Toe - Heel

The Foot and Ankle

Inspection from the front

Deformity

Coronal plane deformity of the knee and ankle such as varus or valgus. Define foot and ankle deformity in terms of pes planovalgus or pes cavovarus. Be very clear in terminology and know what each term means precisely. Talipes equinovarus and calcaneovalgus are often used indiscriminately. Look for torsion of the tibia and femur and any signs of previous trauma. Describe the hindfoot, midfoot and forefoot individually. Is there metatarsus adductus, or a skew foot with hindfoot valgus and midfoot adductus with valgus forefoot? Look for hallux valgus, dorsal bunions ie osteophytes over the metatarsophalangeal joint in hallux rigidus. Lesser toe deformity such as hammer, mallet, claw or simply curly. Congenital features such as syndactily, short toe in brachymetatarsia. Any asymmetry in the feet should lead you to exclude a spinal disorder. Foot shape varies with race but most patterns are that of a Greek foot with a short first ray and an Egyptian foot with a long first ray relative to the second. Note the deformity in hallux valgus with pronation of the hallux, metatarsus primus varus and a prominent medial eminence.

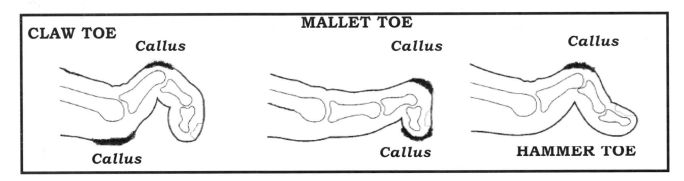

Skin

Loss of skin hair and dry skin with nail dystrophy may be seen in peripheral vascular disease, varicose veins. Skin incisions in the foot and ankle heal very well normally and unless looked for may be missed. Ulcers over bony prominences may be an indicator of vascular problems. Callosities on the dorsum over the interphalangeal joints indicate abnormal pressure with rubbing of shoes. Abnormal nails may indicate a systemic disorder such as pitting in psoriasis.

Contours

Look for any swellings over medial eminence of hallux, fifth toe bunionette, navicular. Ganglions are often seen on the dorsum of the foot. Midfoot arthritis may often lead to a prominent osteophyte over the Chopart or Lisfranc joints.

Wasting

Look for quadriceps and calf muscle wasting. Asymmetry in the feet with clawing on one side should lead you to consider spinal conditions. Wasting of extensor digitorum brevis may be an early sign of a neurological condition. In HSMN the anterolateral muscles are often wasted, leading to an inverted champagne or stork type legs.

The Foot and Ankle

Inspection from the side

Deformity

Look for an equinus posture of the foot which may follow an ankle injury or in post traumatic arthritis. Often the whole limb is held forward compared to the normal side to accommodate for the equinus deformity. In leg length discrepancy the shorter foot is often in equinus and hindfoot in varus to artificially lengthen the length of the limb. A fixed flexion deformity of the knee may lead to an equinus deformity of the foot. The medial longitudinal arch is inspected for pes planus or cavus. As a rough estimate if the thumb can be passed under the arch upto the fifth metatarsal base then a cavus foot exist or if you cannot even start to push your thumb then a pes planus exist. Look at the hindfoot, midfoot and forefoot together when a pes plano valgus foot is present. A midfoot break may occur at Chopart or Lisfranc joints when there are traumatic or degenerate changes accounting for a planus foot.

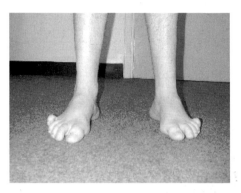

Fig 121. Pes cavovarus foot.

Skin

Look for scars, sinuses, ulcers.

Contours

Swelling around the tuberosity of the navicular tendon e.g. tibialis posterior tendon. The base of fifth metatarsal in overloading of the lateral foot column in pes cavovarus feet.

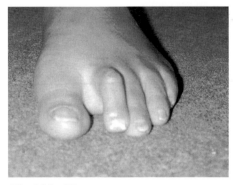

Fig 122. Hammer.

Wasting

Look for wasting of the calf and intrinsic muscles.

The Foot and Ankle

Inspections from behind

Deformity

Normally the heel is in 5-10 degrees of valgus compared to the tibia. This can be determined by drawing a line along the achilles tendon and heel. The angle is increased in a valgus foot and decreased in a varus foot. In a normal foot only the fourth and fifth toes are seen. In a pes planovalgus foot the "too many toe sign" occurs when the second or third toes are also seen. In metatarsus adductus the opposite occurs with the hallux and second toe are seen on the tibial side.
A prominent posterolateral tuberosity of the calcaneum is seen in a Haglund`s deformity and this may have an overlying bursitis.

Skin

Look for scars and sinuses.

Contour

Is there any asymmetry in the calf muscles with wasting in disuse, or in a neurological condition or hypertrophy in a dystrophy? Look fro swelling in the Achilles tendon. Is this at the insertion or more proximal ? Insertional tendonitis occurs in non-rheumatoid inflammatory arthropathy and also in gout. Non insertional swelling may be due to a paratendonopathy or a tendonopathy.

Wasting

Look for wasting of the calf muscles and the hamstrings. In polio the calf muscles are wasted whereas in HSMN the anterolateral muscles are often wasted.

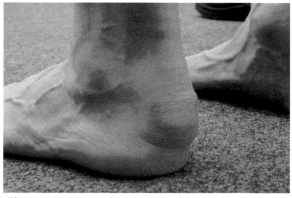

Figure 123. Insertional tendonitis

Gait

Watch the patient walk on level ground and if possible climbing stairs. During gait the information available to the naked eye can be overwhelming. Break each component down beginning by looking at the normal side first. Try to assess each part of the gait cycle and watch the three rockers, heel strike, second rocker and push off. Does the patient strike the floor with the heel or the forefoot first as in a foot drop gait? The heel normally strikes the floor in varus and quickly becomes valgus then finally varus.In a stiff ankle the second rocker is diminished and you may see an early heel raise and absent second rocker. If hallux rigidus or valgus is present, then the third rocker may be affected.
Observe if the midfoot collapses in the stance phase or if the patient weight bears on the outer border in a cavus foot.

Foot and Ankle Examination

Inspection with the patient facing the wall

Double limb heel raise

Make sure that the patient doesn not perform a trick movement by holding onto the door handle or chair. With the hands on a wall at shoulder height, ask the patient to stand on tip toes. Normally the windlass mechanism leads to hindfoot varus, reconstitution of the medal arch and external rotation of the tibia. Conditions that limit this include muscle weakness, subtalar arthritis or coalition, tibialis posterior dysfunction. Frequently forefoot pain and ankle pain may limit this manoeuvre.

Single limb heel raise

Ask the patient to repeat the heel raise by lifting the opposite leg clear off the ground and then standing on tip toe. Early tibialis dysfunction may be detected by this manoeuvre especially if repeated several times.

Inspection with the patient supine on the couch/bed

Skin

Look for areas of high pressure load with callosity. Know the difference between plantar verruca and calluses. Verrucas tend to occur on non weight bearing areas. Calluses may be localised to one metatarsal or diffuse in central metatarsalgia. Calluses may occur on the tips of toes in mallet deformity. Plantar fibroma may be seen in the plantar fascia. Athlete's feet and soft corns between the toes should be inspected for. Ulcers commonly occur in diabetic feet or in peripheral vascular disease. Diabetic foot ulcers occur in high areas subject to high loads. Plantar scars are particularly hard to see once healed, therefore look carefully.

Contour

Look for swellings along the plantar fascia such as fibroma.

Wasting

Wasting of the intrinsics is difficult to see, but look at the fullness medially and laterally over abductor hallucis and digiti minimi.Is there any heel pad or forefoot metatarsal pad atrophy ?

"LOOK - FEEL - MOVE"

FEEL

Start in a systematic way.hindfoot, midfoot then forefoot.

Palpate bony landmarks and around joints.

Hindfoot:	Malleoli. Ankle joint anteriorly, medial and laterally and posterolateral and posteromedial. Feel Tendo Achilles. Is there swelling and tenderness.
Midfoot:	Feel navicular and fifth metatarsal tuberosity.Feel each bone in turn talus, calcaneum, navicular, cuneiforms, and metatarsal. Prominent osteophyte may be felt over arthritic joints.
Forefoot:	Feel each toe phalanx and locate any points of pain. Any bony prominences to account for corns and calluses?

Foot and Ankle Examination

Move

Active range of movement.

Ask the patient to dorsiflex and plantar flex the ankle. (passively). Compare both sides and note any subtle changes. Gross ankle movements are complex and plantar flexion is a composite of supination, adduction and plantarflexion. Dorsflexion is a composite movement also of pronation, abduction and dorsiflexion.

1. Compare movement of ankle range of movement.

2. Midfoot: Ask to invert and evert foot.

3. Forefoot: Ask to dorsi and plantar flex toes and compare sides.

Passive range of movement.

Hindfoot

    Ankle: Assess tibiotalar movement. Put finger and thumb over talar neck and hand over foot as shown. Normal range 10-20 degrees dorsiflexion and 40-55 degrees plantar flexion. (Fig. 124)

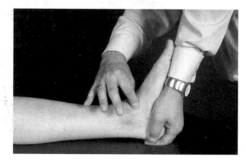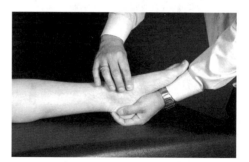

Fig. 124 Ankle ROM.

    Subtalar: With a similar manoeuvre hold talar neck and move the calcaneum from inversion to eversion. Normal range 20-30 degrees inversion and 5-10 degrees eversion. Note any crepitus, pain. (Fig. 125)

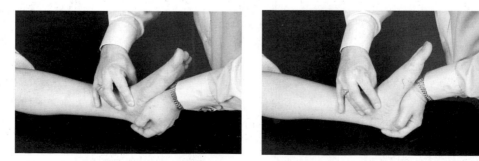

Fig. 125 Subtalar ROM.

Foot and Ankle Examination

Midfoot Chopart: Holding calcaneum, assess midfoot abduction and adduction and rotation. (Fig. 126)

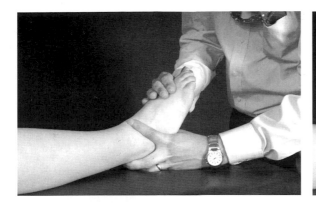
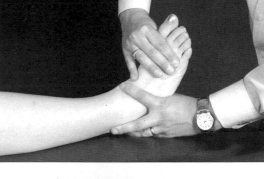
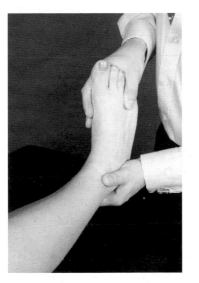
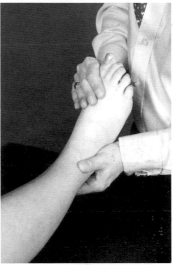

Fig. 126

Lisfranc: Assess saggital plane movement which is minimal for the medial column (TMT 1-3) compared to the lateral column (TMT 4/5) (Fig.127)

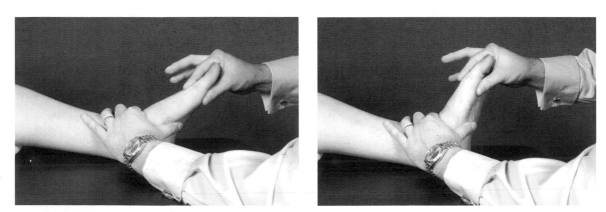

Fig. 127

Foot and Ankle Examination

Forefoot

Hallux   MTP range dorsiflexion 70-90 degrees and 60-90 degrees plantar flexion.
Note any impingement, pain, crepitus. Correct hallux valgus before assessing range.
IP Plantar flexion 70-90 degrees. Dorsiflexion 0-20 degrees. (Fig. 128)

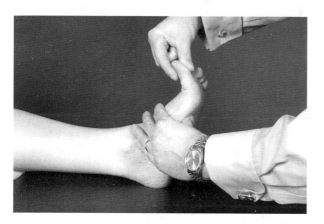 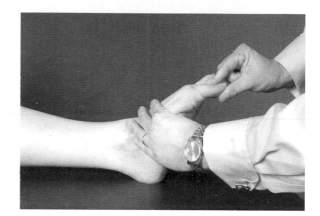

Fig. 128

Lesser toes   MTP up to 90 degrees dorsiflexion and 70 plantarflexion.
IP dorsiflexion 0 degrees, plantarflexion up to 80 degrees.
Note and fixed or flexible deformity.

Tendons   Assess each tendon but testing to resistance. Look and feel tendon and grade strength according
to MRC scale.

Tibialis anterior

Tibialis posterior

EDL

EHL

TA   Silverskiold test

Peroneal longus

Peroneal brevis

Flexor digitorum longus

Foot and Ankle Examination

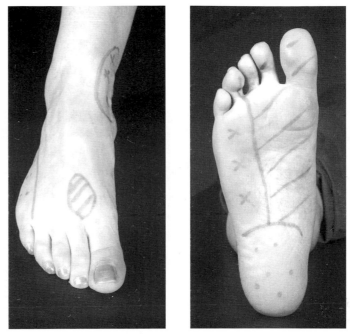

Nerve
Saphenous
Superficial Peroneal
Sural
Deep peroneal
(Fig. 129)

Fig. 129

Plantar medial and lateral nerves.
  Special touch, vibration and Semmes Weinstein monofilament Pulses
  DP and PT

Special Test

Ankle Ligaments

Lateral   Anterior drawer, Inversion compare sides. (Fig. 130)
Medial   Deltoid insufficiency

Instability First TMT   Lachman test AP drawer test
MTP joints   Lachman like test

Syndesmosis   External rotation and squeeze test

Peroneal subluxation/dislocation

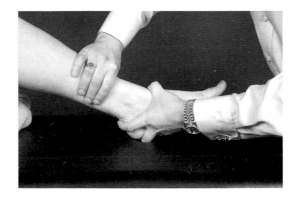

Fig. 130

Foot and Ankle Examination

Nerve

Morton's click. Only positive if it reproduces pain and symptoms. (Fig. 131).

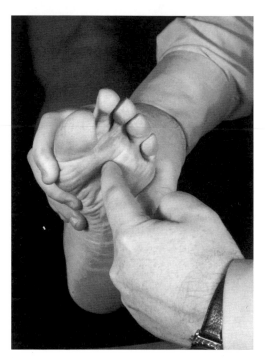

Fig. 131 The Squeeze Test for a Morton's Neuroma typically in the interspace of the third and forth toes.

Coleman block test. (Fig. 132)

To assess subtalar joint movement, if hindfoot moves into valgus when 1st ray drops, then hindfoot is mobile.

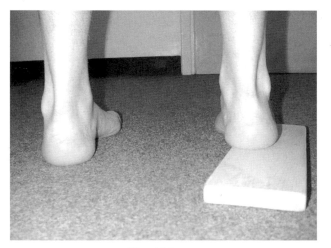

Fig. 132

Tendo achilles
　　Prone.　Arc sign